Health surveys in practice and in potential: a critical review of their scope and methods

ANN CARTWRIGHT

King Edward's Hospital Fund for London

© Crown copyright 1983
First paperback edition 1986
Reprinted 1988
Typeset by Rowland Phototypesetting Limited
Bury St Edmunds, Suffolk
Printed in England by Hollen Street Press Limited
Distributed for the King's Fund by Oxford University Press

ISBN 0 19 724639 7

King's Fund Publishing Office
14 Palace Court
London W2 4HT

Contents

Tables

Figure

Acknowledgements

One very pleasant aspect of working on this review has been the generous way in which people have given me their time, their ideas and access to their papers. Those who have done so include: Abe Adelstein, Rob Anderson, Jean Aitken-Swan, Sara Arber, Grace Barrs, Mel Bartley, Toni Belfield, Geoff Beltram, Val Beral, Mildred Blaxter, Ann Bowling, John Brotherston, Vera Carstairs, May Clarke, Brendan Devlin, Mollie Dixon, Robin Dowie, Michael D'Souza, Karen Dunnell, Mary Durant, David Fruin, Eileen Goddard, Phoebe Hall, Austin Heady, Lisbeth Hockey, Tim Holt, Raymond Illsley, Margot Jefferys, John Knowelden, Joyce Leeson, John McEwan, Sally Macintyre, Fred Martin, Louis Moss, Ann Oakley, Donald Patrick, Hedley Peach, Sheila Pease, Aly Rashid, Martin Richards, Ian Russell, Billie Shepperdson, Madeleine Simms, Alwyn Smith, Christopher Smith, Gordon Smith, Marguerite Smith, Thelma Thomas, Barbara Thompson, Martin Vessey, Mike Wadsworth, Michael Warren and Frank Whitehead.

I am sorry I have not been able to take up all their comments and suggestions.

In addition the librarians at the London School of Hygiene, the Office of Population Censuses and Surveys, the Royal Free Hospital and the Royal Society of Medicine have been extremely helpful. I have been ably supported by Irene Browne, Anne Fleissig and Ann Jacoby who checked the report, André Simonoviescz who did the proof reading and Carol Potter the reproducing. Irene Browne also typed the various drafts with great speed and accuracy.

The review was funded by the Social Science Research Council and the Department of Health and Social Security.

I am grateful to them all.

Foreword

I was first asked to do this critical review by the Statistics Committee of the SSRC who, as I understand it, wanted a discussion of both the contents and methods of surveys in the health and health care field. The members hoped that this discussion would lead to a more critical awareness of the potentialities, limitations and pitfalls of survey methods and to the identification of subject areas that might usefully be explored in the future. Clearly it was an ambitious project and the two months' consultantship that the SSRC could fund was inadequate to do it in any depth. Fortunately the DHSS were prepared to fund the project jointly with SSRC and for a somewhat longer period.

The project appealed to me because I am interested in both the subject matter and the methodology of health surveys. It was also an opportunity to take time out from the business of carrying out such surveys, to consider, in a wider perspective, what surveys were doing and how they were being done. For many years I had been immersed in the process of running a small research unit, obtaining funds, developing proposals, matching projects and people, organising surveys and writing them up. Here was a chance to stop for a short while and think about what my colleagues in the same field and I had been doing over the years. I hoped too that this would suggest appropriate directions for future work.

It was a larger and more difficult task than I had realised. To do it justice would require years rather than months. And I had problems with the nature of the task. Although it seems to make sense to review methods alongside the aims, I began to feel quite schizophrenic about it. At one point I would be immersed in the purpose and the results of a study, and at another fascinated by the techniques. This conflict is I think inherent in the nature of the task and could not be resolved by adopting a different structure. Initially I had intended to use a frame based more on the methods than on the subject areas. But I was persuaded that it was more appropriate to start with the themes of the studies, and I think this is right: methods usually depend on aims, not the other way round.

An initial uncertainty was about the audience for this review. The one I would *like* to attract consists of five groups: 1 people doing, or thinking of doing, survey research in the health field; 2 teachers of survey methods, particularly those teaching people likely to be working in the health field; 3 the people in a position to commission such research – and those involved in that process; 4 editors and publishers who take part, or might take part, in the dissemination of research findings; and 5 practitioners, administrators and consumers who might make use of such research. (Practitioners and administrators are targets for a further reason: they can facilitate the access of researchers to records and samples.) It is ambitious to try to attract such a wide and varied audience. Those who carry out such research will I hope be tempted to read about themselves from the idiosyncratic perspective of one of their colleagues. Those in other categories may feel somewhat daunted at the prospect of ploughing through such a lengthy and at times fairly technical and detailed report. But if survey research is to be appropriately funded and used it is important that those funding and using it and those disseminating the results should be able to distinguish good studies from bad and this depends on some knowledge of the limitations and the pitfalls of survey research. People may be more inclined to read about technical problems in practice than in theory. Some may be interested in a particular subject area and prepared to read a chapter on that. Others may be more attracted to the chapter on methodological issues and want to start with that, so I have provided references back to the earlier chapters if they should wish to pursue particular points. In one way or another I hope to attract the main target groups for this review: those directly involved in the initiation, sponsorship, practice and teaching of this type of research, and those who might make use of or disseminate its findings.

1 *Introduction*

In this review I outline some of the ways in which surveys have contributed and could contribute further to the understanding of health and health care. It is a review of the range of subject areas covered by surveys in the health field and of the variety of methods that have been used to illuminate them. I have taken as my starting point the different types of questions addressed by surveys in this area and have illustrated them by surveys which have adopted different sorts of methodological approaches. In the discussion of the studies I try to show how the different aspects of survey methodology relate to the usefulness and limitations of the surveys.

Structure and scope of the review

Surveys are essentially a research tool by which facts can be ascertained, theories confirmed or refuted, ideas explored and values identified and illuminated. So the sorts of questions with which the surveys are concerned relate to the distribution and association of facts and attitudes. In the health field surveys can contribute to the identification or description and measurement or analysis of: 1 health and illness, 2 the nature of disease, 3 needs for different sorts of care, 4 factors associated with the use of services, 5 the effects of care, 6 acceptability of care and 7 the organisation of care. So these are the broad headings under which different types of surveys are considered in this review. Quality of care is not considered separately because surveys assess quality by seeing to what extent needs are met, services used effectively, outcomes of care are good, care is acceptable and organisation efficient and effective.

Methodological issues are also discussed under these headings and most of the chapters have both a methodological and a subject-related conclusion. The methodological issues are also brought together for a wider discussion in a penultimate chapter, and the ethics and use of surveys explored at the end.

One problem arising from this structure is that many surveys cover a range of problems and attempt to answer different types of questions. But as I have focused on a particular subject I have tended to concentrate on one aspect of these multi-purpose studies. Thus in discussing the Survey of Sickness and the General Household Survey I have been concerned mainly with their measures of health and sickness and have only considered their data on the use of services when they illuminate the findings on health and sickness. This means that my assessments of these multi-purpose studies are limited to the contribution they make to the area under which I have discussed them.

Another complication is the variation in the detail with which different studies have been discussed, and therefore in the emphasis put on them. In the earlier chapters I have tended to discuss methods in detail, in later ones I have only described unusual or innovative methods or dealt with methodological aspects that have not already been considered.

This review is illustrative and not in any way comprehensive. Alderson and Dowie (1979) did a comprehensive review of health surveys and related studies in the United Kingdom up to 1976 and I have drawn on this. Like them I have confined the studies I discuss in any detail to those done in the United Kingdom and there is some similarity in the structures of our two reviews although the emphasis is different. We both have sections on needs and on use of services but whereas they discuss the use of different types of services I consider the questions that surveys on use are attempting to answer. They have a comparatively short chapter on the evaluation of medical care whereas I have two chapters related to the effects of care and the acceptability of services. This different emphasis arises because they were concerned with all the studies that have been done whereas I am concerned with gaps as well as achievement and am able to devote more space to the discussion of a single survey in an unusual field and to ignore many studies that have been done in roughly similar fields.

Ideally the chance of a survey being included in this review would be inversely related to the number of studies in that field and to the number using those particular techniques – the more innovatory, both in relation to subject and methods, the higher the likelihood of it being included. In practice the selection has been decidedly biased. Within the subject and method categories I have discussed studies I know about with reports that are easily available to me, so my own studies are over-represented. What I have *not* done is to select studies deliberately because I felt their methods were good or bad. For the most part I did not know enough about them to assess their quality until I started to consider them in detail.

Some definitions

Platt (1978) described a survey in these terms: 'a technique of data collection, that is the systematic and structured questioning, either by interview or by questionnaire, of a relatively large number of respondents'. This is a useful operational definition for the purpose of this review even though it leaves the 'relatively large number of respondents' undefined. It clearly *excludes* studies of records and observational techniques, although I will consider these as ways of validating survey techniques and show how a combination of a survey approach and studies based on records or observations can be rewarding in certain situations. It does not specify the way in which respondents are selected so surveys of consecutive cases are covered as well as random* samples of different populations. I have however confined the review to surveys of people selected in some sort of systematic way. My other reservation about Platt's definition relates to 'the systematic and structured questioning'; most of the studies I discuss conform to this definition but some which use unstructured questionnaires are also included.

Another term which should be discussed at this stage is health. For many of the studies that are included, sickness is a more appropriate term. But health is wider and the review will encompass surveys of childbearing and of contraception which fall within the wider field of health and health care. However I have not ventured into the areas of mental illness, psychiatric care or 'positive health' because I have no knowledge or experience in those fields.

---

* Random is used here in the statistical sense so that a random sample is one in which each member of the defined population has a defined, and usually an equal, chance of being included.

2 General measures of health and sickness

There are a number of reasons for seeking general measures of health and sickness. It is helpful to be able to make comparisons over time so that we can evaluate the effect of changing services or of changing circumstances that may be associated with the prevalence of ill-health. Such measures can also make it possible to compare the needs of different geographical areas or of people in different social groups. They could contribute greatly to our ability to plan services effectively and allocate resources appropriately.

A traditional measure of health status was mortality, and indeed standardised mortality ratios, along with other indices, are still used, at the recommendation of the Resource Allocation Working Party, to determine revenue targets for Regional Health Authorities, (DHSS 1976). But as a *Lancet* editorial in 1981 put it 'counting the dead is not enough' and Martini et al (1977) have demonstrated that measures of mortality are too insensitive to medical care to be useful in evaluating health services in developed countries.

So people have turned to surveys for general measures of health and sickness. And since the purpose of these measures is to make comparisons such surveys tend to be ongoing ones, carried out on comparable samples at different points in time over a number of years. In addition, and again for comparative purpose, such surveys usually collect information about use of services and about incapacity. Two national studies of this nature covering England and Wales have been the Survey of Sickness and the General Household Survey.

In this chapter I describe these two surveys, some of the ways in which they have been used, and then I discuss the limitations and the potential of continuing health surveys in the measurement of health and sickness. After that I describe briefly another approach which uses perceived health status as a prediction of the need for and use of health services: the Nottingham health profile.

The Survey of Sickness

This study started during the war in 1943. It was initiated because of food rationing, long hours of work, general stress and anxiety and the deleterious effects these were expected to have on health (Logan and

Brooke 1957). In fact, as Logan and Brooke point out, vital statistics showed that 1942 was a record breaking year: maternal and infant mortality rates, the proportion of still births and the standardised death rate among civilians were the lowest ever recorded in England and Wales. Incidence of notifiable infectious diseases was also remarkably low. But such statistics did not reveal details of the 'national well or ill-being' since minor ailments and the 'below par' feeling did not come within their scope. Reports of crowded surgeries and hospital out-patient departments had raised anxieties about the nation's health.

The study was carried out by the Wartime (later the Government) Social Survey, now the Social Survey division of the Office of Population Censuses and Surveys.* Within that organisation the survey was known as the Health Index. It was continued until 1952, four years after the introduction of the NHS. Random samples of the adult population were selected each month and questioned about their health in the two or three preceding calendar months. Some of the methods used and the variations in them are shown in Table 1.

The questions started with a general one on health: 'How was your

Table 1   The Survey of Sickness: variations in methods

Sampling frame:	National Register 1943–1951 covered all residents
	Electoral register 1951–1952 excluded aliens
Ages covered:	16–64 1943–1944
	16 and over December 1944–1951
	21 and over 1951–1952
Number interviewed each month:	2,500 initially
	3,000 ⎫
	4,000 ⎭ at later stages
Period asked about:	previous three months 1943–1949 June
	previous two months 1949 July–1952
Questions asked:	'anything wrong with your nerves' added to check list of symptoms relating to September, October, November, 1945 onwards
Classification of illness:	MRC Provisional Classification 1943–1948
	International Statistical Classification 1949–1952

* For convenience I have referred to it throughout as the Government Social Survey.

general health during _____ (study months)?' This was followed by a broad one about ill-health: 'Did you have any illness, ailment, poisoning or injury of any kind or trouble with long standing complaints during _____?' Finally there was a more specific one: 'Have you had anything wrong in the way of colds, catarrh, or nose and throat trouble or anything wrong with your eyes, ears, teeth, headpains, chest, heart, stomach or indigestion, liver, kidneys, bowels or constipation, legs, feet, hands, arms or rheumatism, skin complaints, infectious diseases or anything wrong with your nerves?' To all women – 'Have you had anything wrong in the way of women's complaints?'

For the most part this check list relates to parts of the body – nose, eyes, ears, chest, heart, legs, feet, skin, and so on – rather than symptoms or conditions. The exceptions to this are colds, catarrh, indigestion, constipation, rheumatism and infectious diseases. I have not found a statement of the rationale behind this but gather it would be along these lines:

1 The initial intention was to ask about parts of the body on the grounds that it was not thought appropriate to ask people to make diagnoses.
2 To stimulate people to think about their health problems, and to try to avoid bias the various parts of the body were specified in turn from top to toe.
3 A symptom 'headpains' was included because to ask if people had anything wrong with their head might be misunderstood.
4 Other symptoms such as colds, catarrh and indigestion were included to give an indication of the level of sickness the survey was intended to cover.
5 Rheumatism was included because it was found that once this diagnosis had been made, whether by the persons themselves or by their doctors, it ceases to be thought of as something wrong with a particular part of the body. People fail to recognise their rheumatism in a question about legs, feet, hands or arms.

In my view the most notable omission from the list is the back or backache. And I feel that so many modifications need to be made to a list of parts of the body that it would be more appropriate to start with a list of symptoms (See Cartwright 1959a). People were also asked about incapacity and medical consultations and data about age, occupation and income were recorded. It was recognised (Logan and

Brooke 1957) that there was some lack of clarity over incapacity rates because of dual definitions applied to persons at work and those not at work, while over medical consultations it was uncertain whether those taking place in hospital were intended to be included or excluded.

The data from the Survey of Sickness were analysed along medical lines: mean month's sickness, prevalence, incapacity and consultation rates were computed; each condition was coded by General Register Office staff according to the MRC's classification of diseases and injuries. (Later the International Classification of Diseases was used.) For publication purposes two breakdowns by type of condition were used: a short one of 18 selected diagnoses ranging from tuberculosis of the lungs, ulcer of the stomach and duodenum, and psychoneurosis, mental disorders (the three least common ones) to colds and influenza, rheumatism and ill-defined conditions (the most common); and a longer list of 100 causes covering pneumonia; pleurisy, emphysema and lung abscess; and cellulitis and lymphanginitis at its most esoteric; and common colds, headaches and nervousness and debility at the other end of the scale.

Ingenious assessments were made of the reliability of this material by comparing the prevalence of gastric duodenal and anastomatic ulcers with data from the Ministry of Food for priority milk allowances, while the amount of pernicious anaemia reported was compared with mortality rates taking account of the changing survival due to the introduction of liver therapy (Stocks 1949).

The survey was clearly based on a medical model. Logan and Brooke (1957) saw its two main defects as its use of non-medical statements and its dependence upon the memory of the persons interviewed. But they regarded it as 'an important contribution towards the methodology of morbidity enumeration' and felt it 'amply repaid the relatively modest amount of time, trouble and expense it entailed.'

Stocks (1949) on the other hand emphasised the advantages of a survey that covered a random sample of the population. 'Only 23% of people recording an illness or injury during a month had consulted a doctor during that month and this . . . suggests that any system of national morbidity statistics based on doctors' own records could not provide a complete picture of the illness occurring.'

The methodological aspect of the Survey of Sickness which attracted great attention was the problem of memory errors. This was analysed by Stocks (1949) Gray (1955) Slater (1946) as well as Logan and Brooke (1957). When discussing the methods and results of the

Survey, Logan and Brooke comment: 'In any future survey of sickness the effect of memory error would be reduced by shortening the period enquired about.' But while they were aware of at least some of the deficiencies in the interview data they did not appear to recognise all the limitations in the statistical analyses. Presenting data on sickness and prevalence rates by income group and pointing out the higher rates in lower income groups they draw attention to: 1 the high refusal rate to the question on income, 2 the fact that a person may be in a low income group because he is ill, 3 since the income group relates to the 'chief wage earner' or 'head of household' the number of people in the family should be taken into account. They did not point out that income is related to age so that any meaningful comparison should be standardised by age.

One basic methodological implication from the comparisons with data from other sources made by Stocks (1949) – that reliable data on certain medical issues can be obtained from surveys of the population – was not generally accepted by the medical profession. Because of this the Survey of Sickness was little used. Although one of the main findings of the survey was the iceberg of ill-health in the community which did not reach the doctor, Morris (1957) in his book *Uses of Epidemiology* made no reference to it, or use of its data. But his discussion (page 44) of the iceberg phenomenon would have been strengthened by reference to the survey's findings. Neither did sociologists exploit its potential. Titmuss (1968) in a discussion of the way the higher income groups make better use of the Health Service, made no use of information from the Survey of Sickness, although he referred to some much less convincing data in support of his argument (See Cartwright and O'Brien 1976). Historians too ignored it. Lindsey (1962) in *Socialized medicine in England and Wales: the National Health Service 1948–61*, a book that claimed to be 'an authoritative work that people could approach without a feeling that the author was twisting the facts or witholding important data to prove a thesis', makes no reference to it.

McKeown and Lowe (1966) quoted its findings and emphasised what now seem to be commonplace results. In *An Introduction to social medicine* (page 45) they comment:

'There are obvious weaknesses in morbidity statistics based on what a person remembers and is prepared to tell a non-medical interviewer about recent ill-health; nevertheless they provide useful information that cannot be obtained in any other way. Two out of three persons reported an awareness of some ill-health during the month before the interview, and, as expected, awareness of ill-health increased steeply with age. Less expected was the finding that at all ages females complained of more ill-health than males.'

Perhaps the most important findings from the Survey of Sickness relate to trends over time since it covered the period from the middle of the war to after the introduction of the National Health Service. To quote Logan and Brooke again: 'The first twelve months of the new Service must be fitted into the general pattern of trends and it then becomes apparent that there was an increase in medical consultation rates among women aged 16–44 and people of 65 and over . . . The trend of the figures suggests that the increase in consultation rates among women and old people was due to their now being more ready to consult a doctor when sick than they had been prior to July 1948.' In the light of this I find their concluding discussion of the Survey of Sickness somewhat surprising: 'The survey method has established itself as a valuable technique in various fields, and it has its place as a method of morbidity ascertainment. It can best make its contribution however, not as a permanent operation designed to measure the total load of ill-health, its nature, distribution and trends, but to contribute, from time to time as the need arises, particular items of information on illness and its effects that cannot be readily obtained in a routine way.'

The *British Medical Journal* was more positive. In a leader (1946) 'Are the people more healthy?' it described the Survey of Sickness as 'a direct estimation of the sickness experience of the nation' and went on to advocate: 'If in peacetime far larger samples of the population could be investigated . . . then the survey started during the war should bring in more and more useful returns, and enable those in charge of, or working in, the Health Service to get a much more accurate measure of the health of the people than has been possible in the past. What we want is more information and less propaganda.'

But the cuts in government spending in 1952 meant the end of the Survey of Sickness. To me it seems a pity that economies were not made in a more discriminating way. I would question the need for the survey to have continued on the same scale and at such frequent intervals and with the detailed medical coding. But a series of regular, possibly quarterly, studies of illness and consultation rates on somewhat smaller samples could have heightened awareness of both geographical and social inequalities which might in turn have led to a more appropriate distribution of services. However even continuous surveys suffer from a number of disadvantages when making comparisons over time. These will be discussed after the other British study which collects health data on a continuing basis has been described.

The General Household Survey

This study, which started in 1971, is not confined to health and health services. Indeed it was conceived as a 'co-operative research service' meeting a variety of needs within one survey framework 'to develop a government research instrument which could examine the way in which different policy areas interacted' (OPCS 1973). In relation to health the original interest in the GHS was as 'a vehicle to monitor the use of health and social services in relation to some of the other personal and household data collected in the survey. This was broadly intended to cover the extent to which members of households are unable to carry out their normal activities through illness or disability and to what extent they make use of the health and social services to help them return to normal activities. At a relatively late stage in the development of the survey . . . it was suggested . . . that an attempt should be made to establish the illness or disability which prevented normal activities.'

The sampling unit for the GHS is addresses. From 1971–1974 a three-stage rotating sample design was used, but a change in sample design in January 1975 was made necessary by the reorganisation of local government in Britain. Since then a two stage design has been used with electoral wards as the primary sampling units. Published response rates relate to households not individuals. In 1978 71% of households cooperated completely, all adult members (aged 16 or more) of the households answering the questions, 85% responded at least partially – some or all members cooperating.

The only questions in the health, or rather sickness, field to be included throughout the 1971–78 period related to use of services: to general practitioner consultations and outpatient attendances. Some questions on chronic sickness or chronic health problems and on acute sickness or short term health problems were included throughout the period, but the questions were changed radically in 1977 and those on chronic sickness were also amended between 1971 and 1972 and during 1973. The rationale for the 1977 changes was this: 'From 1971–76 the main emphasis . . . was on establishing patterns of service use in relation to chronic and acute sickness and the wide range of demographic information collected by the GHS . . . As expected, the survey showed that changes in the health of the population were taking place slowly, and by 1976 it was clear that in the next few years little extra information of value would be gained by further repeating the same series of questions . . . In 1977, therefore, a different approach was used, in which more emphasis was placed on respondents' own perceptions of their state of health . . . the effect of health problems on people's lives and how people cope with ill-health . . . A major departure from the method of questioning used in previous years was that, as part of the initial questions used to establish the presence or absence of ill-health, respondents were shown check lists of common health problems or symptoms.'*

The questions on acute sickness or short term health problems also changed in 1977. Between 1971–76 informants were asked: 'During the two weeks which ended last Sunday, did you (or any of your children under 15) have to cut down at all on things you usually do because of (this illness/disability or some other) illness or injury?' From 1977 the question was: 'I'd now like to ask about anything (else) you've had the matter with you in the 14 days ending yesterday.' A check list was used, this one relating mainly to symptoms.**

Because of the new focus on the subjective views of people's state of health, information about the health of children under 16 was not obtained although data about their use of services were continued.

The revised questions tapped a very different level of response. In 1977, 56% of men and 70% of women reported chronic health problems whereas before that about a quarter of men and women said they had a long standing illness. And in 1976 only 8.7% of adult males

* In relation to chronic problems these were bronchitis; arthritis or rheumatism; sciatica, lumbago or recurring backache; persistent skin trouble (e.g. eczema); asthma; hay fever; recurring stomach trouble; being constipated all or most of the time; piles; blood pressure; heart trouble; persistent foot trouble (e.g. bunions, ingrowing toe nails); trouble with varicose veins; nervous trouble or persistent depression; diabetes; persistent trouble with gums or mouth; (trouble or pain with periods/menopause/the change).

** A cough, catarrh or phlegm; diarrhoea; heartburn, wind or indigestion; shortness of breath; dizziness or giddiness; earache or discomfort in the ears; swollen ankles; nervy, tense or depressed; a cold or flu; a sore throat; difficulty in sleeping; pains in the chest; a backache or pains in the back; nausea or vomiting; feeling tired for no apparent reason; rashes, itches or other skin trouble; toothache or trouble with gums.'

and 10.2% of adult females reported restricted activity in the two week reference period while in 1977 32% of adult males, 38% of adult females said they did something differently from usual in the 14 days before interview because of short term health problems. Other health related topics included in the GHS in some years up to 1979 were health in general in the previous 12 months, (1977–79), help from people outside the household with housework or shopping (1971–74), access to general practitioners (1977), appointments with OP departments (1973–76), inpatient spells (1971–76), use of health and welfare services (1971–76), hearing and sight (1977–79), medicine taking (1973), smoking (1972–76 and 1978). More recently, in 1982, it has covered use of private medical services and insurance for private medical care.

The inclusion of different topics may influence responses to some of the continuing general questions about sickness. For example, in 1973 the series of questions on health started with one about different types of medicines that had been taken 'during the seven days ending yesterday'. Thinking about this could change people's level of awareness about their health during this time so that a later question about restriction in activities in 'the two weeks ending last Sunday' could be affected either because of a change in threshold or because of some confusion over the different periods that were being asked about.

Another methodological problem arises in relation to children since parents provide data for all their children. In large families parents may be both less aware of and less likely to report relatively minor conditions. And since family size is related to socio-economic group this may be a source of systematic distortion in these analyses. Some data illustrating this are given in a study by Blaxter and Paterson, 1982, page 41.

Turning to the use that has been made of the health or sickness data from the GHS, several people have related these data to socio-economic group and to consultation rates in attempts to understand the relationship between the three variables.

Forster (1976) used the 1971 and 1972 GHS data to analyse social class differences in sickness and general practitioner consultations. He used age standardised rates and concluded that 'the apparent advantages of the higher consultation rates in the lower social groups . . . are eliminated or reversed when morbidity is also considered'. Similarly the Black report (DHSS 1980) on *Inequalities in Health* concludes (page 100) that despite 'strong reservations about the restricted nature of the indicators and about fluctuations . . . from year to year . . . the evidence (from the GHS) can be taken to suggest that the level of consultation among partly skilled and unskilled manual workers does not match their need for health care.' Collins and Klein (1980) reached a different conclusion. In their analysis of the 1974 General Household Survey data they looked at the proportion of users of health care services in four groups: the not ill, the acutely sick, the chronically sick without restricted activity and the chronically sick with restricted activity, and state 'contrary to the conclusions of existing publications, the analysis shows that the NHS has achieved equity in terms of access of primary health care: there is no consistent bias against the lower socio-economic groups'.

The different conclusions reached by Forster, the Black report and by Collins and Klein stem in part from the different periods they have used for analysis, and the different methods adopted. But I think Collins and Klein go beyond the logical limits of the data.

Scott-Samuel (1981) in a critique of their analyses argues that the question used to classify the 'acutely-sick' does not 'necessarily imply the need for a visit to the general practitioner and cannot therefore be related with any validity to the "use" data. Even if (as is probable) a partial relation exists it could well be subject to a systematic social class bias.' He also contends that the chronic morbidity group could carry a social class bias, and points out that 'despite their acknowledgment that use and need cannot accurately be matched, Collins and Klein go on to match them'.

The data for children present rather different problems. Blaxter (1981) points out (page 118) that there has been 'a very marked deficit' in reported outpatient attendances 'for both male and (especially) female children aged 0–4 in unskilled manual families, when they are compared with all the rest'. She also draws attention (page 102) to the notable sex difference among children – more illness both chronic and acute being reported for boys than girls. Commenting on the social class trend in acute illness rates for boys which go in the opposite direction to those for adults she says 'all the weight of the evidence suggests, however, that [this] is unlikely to be a true tendency and must be affected by mothers' identification or reporting'. She attaches more credence (page 171) to what she describes as the reverse for social class trend for children (especially boys aged 0–4) in general practice consultation rates and says this urgently requires explanation.

Apart from socio-economic variations other findings of note from the GHS health data relate to age, sex and trends over time. GHS data have also been used to make estimates of the prevalence of disability among children (Weale and Bradshaw 1980). These are discussed in Chapter 4.

Collins and Klein's analysis of health and the use of primary care services suggest that the elderly (aged 65 or more) 'often have below average access rates'. They find this surprising 'given the evidence that rationing by queueing tends to encourage use by those whose time costs are lowest'. They conclude 'this might be expected to favour the elderly, so our finding that when sick they are getting at best no more than their share of access may give cause for concern'.

Another finding emphasised by Collins and Klein is that women aged 40–64 make considerably lower demands on primary care than men of the same age. Given the commonly held view that women of this age are relatively heavy users of the service this finding is important.

Some time trends were identified in the OPCS report on the 1976 GHS. This notes that while the questions on chronic health have shown little or no significant change over time, between 1971 and 1976 'there was an increase, ranging from just under a third to nearly two-thirds, in the reported acute sickness rate among children under 15 of both sexes and females aged 15–44'. The GHS report comments that 'it is only possible to speculate that there may be a relationship between the increase in reported acute sickness rates among women aged 15–44 and the increasing tendency for wives and mothers in this age group to go out to work, and that this latter phenomenon may also be associated with the increase in reported acute sickness rates among children. Without further investigation this hypothesis, . . . must remain unsubstantiated at the present time by GHS data.' (OPCS 1978, pages 72–3). It seems strange, in a survey whose raison d'être was to examine the ways in which different policy areas interacted, that this hypothesis could not be tested by further analyses with other GHS data relating to employment!

But in spite of the limitations in the data, as the Black report (page 48) recognises, 'for the analysis of social class and occupational differences in morbidity the only *regular* source of information provided by central government is to be found in the General Household Survey'.

Limitations and potential of continuing health surveys

In discussing the limitations of continuing health surveys it is helpful to distinguish between those limitations which are inevitable and those which relate only to the methods used on particular surveys. As far as the latter are concerned I have confined my comments to the General Household Survey as that is ongoing.

The discussion covers four areas: 1 trends over time, 2 the aims and wording of questions about health, 3 analysis of the data and 4 validation of survey data.

Trends over time Even when similar samples are asked precisely the same questions there are problems in interpreting trends over time. One difficulty is that expectations may change: people who regarded themselves as healthy at one time may have different standards later. Another problem is that changing conditions may complicate the interpretation of trends. For example, there was a decline in home visiting by general practitioners between 1964 and 1977, but over that period there was an increase in the proportion of people using cars to go to their doctor's surgery and those who used cars had fewer home visits than those who went by public transport or walked all the way (see Cartwright and Anderson 1981). So an analysis by home visiting and mode of transport was necessary to see whether or not the decline in home visiting could be attributed to this reason alone, or whether other factors such as changes in health might also have contributed. Such difficulties as these are inevitable complications of continuing series of data whether they are routine service data about use, censuses or surveys.

Even some methodological changes are outside the control of the survey organiser, as for instance when boundary changes affect sampling designs or there is an alteration to eligibility in lists that have been used for sampling frames (for example, when the age at which people were entitled to vote dropped from 21 to 18). But other changes may be initiated by the organisers when they become aware of limitations in their current techniques: they are then faced with a conflict between sacrificing continuity or perpetuating unsatisfactory methods.

If only small changes over time are observed the usefulness of a continuing survey may be questioned and it is tempting to introduce modifications rather than continue to collect the same sort of data and findings. As mentioned earlier this was one reason behind the 1977 changes in the GHS health questions. It might have been more logical from this point of view to conclude that if circumstances are changing slowly surveys are only needed at infrequent intervals. In practice the GHS reverted to many of the earlier questions about health in 1979 so that some comparisons over time could then be made.

Another reason for the 1977 changes was that the proportions reporting illness were small, even though it was known from other studies that much larger proportions were concerned about their health. So what do questions about health attempt to find out and what can they find out?

The aim and wording of questions about health Basically the aim is to make comparisons of relative health or sickness over time or between groups of individuals. The way such comparisons are used is to assess relative need. Various types of need will be discussed in a later chapter. Here I am concerned with the problem of how to ask questions about health that will indicate *relative need* in a way that is independent of the use of health services – that is, so that the measure is not dependent on individuals having contact with the services. In practice it is impossible for an index of relative need to be completely independent of existing services since perceptions of health and sickness as well as any measures or observations will be conditioned to some extent on the services available – or on the absence of such services. But for assessing need the aim must be to minimise that dependence.

Given that the method of obtaining information is by asking questions about health and sickness, not about use of services, there is still a wide range of possibilities from the very general questions about perceptions about state of health as good, fairly good or not good to detailed specific questions about symptoms such as the MRC has developed to establish information about chronic bronchitis. In between there is the possibility of check lists of varying specificity and comprehensiveness. And obviously a survey can include both general and specific questions. But if the survey is to cover all types of ill-health, then it is probably inappropriate to go into much detail about any particular symptom or condition. It would therefore seem that the questions should be designed to make people think about their health and to overcome problems that particular groups in the population may have about expressing their perceptions and experiences. Check lists can be helpful both in stimulating people to think about different aspects of their health and in providing terms in which people can describe their health. People may be hesitant to use what they feel are slang terms to the interviewer while at the same time not being able to think of what they feel would be a more appropriate terminology. The main danger of a check list is that it is likely to create a bias towards the conditions included in it. (It also means that people use the same phrases, but if their reports are classified appropriately this does not matter for the statistical analysis – only for more vivid presentation or more anthropological interests.) So the check list needs to be comprehensive and to use well understood terms and phrases. Methodological studies are needed to ensure that these aims are achieved.

Another function of a check list is to indicate the *level* of ill-health with which the study is concerned. If no indication is given about this some respondents will report colds or headaches, others will not. Whether or not they do so does not necessarily indicate different perceptions about their health, but rather different perceptions about the purpose of the survey.

What of the health questions on the GHS? From 1971–76 the main questions related to 'long-standing illness, disability or infirmity' and restrictions in activities in a two week period due to illness, disability or injury. The argument was that 'although answers to questions about behaviour are subject to environmental influence, they are nevertheless more objective than an informant's opinion about his health state' (OPCS 1973, page 264). I think this is disputable. The concept of 'cutting down on things you usually do' is open to subjective interpretation in much the same way as perceptions about symptoms; and there is the additional problem that having to cut down on things also depends on the level of usual activity. The questions during this period gave no indication of the level of ill-health with which the survey was concerned (what proportion I wonder reported long-standing disabilities with bunions or ingrowing toe nails?), made no attempt to overcome any hesitation or doubts about reporting such things as piles and gave no help in indicating the phrases that might be used to describe problems with conditions like the menopause or mental illness.

In 1977 and 1978 'more emphasis was placed on respondents' own perceptions of their state of health'; check lists were introduced; the questions changed radically as did the amount and probably the level of ill-health that they elicited.

Leaving aside the fact that questions about the health of children were no longer included, I have three criticisms of the 1977–78 health questions in the GHS:

1 A number of the questions about health problems were not independent of what people do about the problems and the use they make of services. Some chronic problems were apparently only identified because people took medicines for them. As the published analyses give no information about how often this happened it is not possible to tell whether it was important numerically, although it is conceptually.

2 The number and complexity of the questions and their dependency make the data hard to use and, I would have thought, tax the concentration, patience and memory of anyone who was old or frail. For example, someone who was not bedfast but had at least one chronic condition and was taking some medicine would have to answer about 90 items of information about their health *before* coming to the details about consultations. And this after they have already been questioned about their household, housing, employment, leisure, education, country of birth and father's occupation. Later they would also be asked about income.

3 The firm division that is made into acute and chronic sickness is unrealistic. This applied both before and after 1977. It seems to me unhelpful to make such a rigid distinction since many conditions do not fit easily into this dichotomy. For chronic conditions the GHS question (in 1977 and 1978) refers to 'health problems that keep recurring or that you have all or most of the time – apart from things like colds or stomach upsets'. Optimists will think a condition they have had a few times is unlikely to recur while pessimists will regard it as likely to do so. There will be differences in the stage at which people with bronchitis or rheumatism or depression recognise or accept that it is something they have all or most of the time. And it may be unkind, as well as, in my view, unnecessary from the viewpoint of the survey, to pose questions which may precipitate the recognition that a complaint is likely to recur or is present most of the time. For some people a chronic condition may have become so much part of themselves or of their lives that they cease to think of it as a health or sickness problem. But questions can overcome this problem without imposing this classification on all conditions. The division into acute and chronic conditions applied to the analyses of the data as well as to the questions asked.

Analysis of the data The published analyses of the GHS data on health have clearly been constrained by space and costs. They are limited and unimaginative and portray little of the wealth of material that has been collected. The major disappointment is in the little use that has been made of data from other sections of the GHS such as housing, migration, education and employment apart from some analyses, in the early 1971–1973 studies, by employment status and job satisfaction. Illustrations of other limitations are:

1 The very broad age groups that are used: 16–44/45–64/65–74/75 +. This makes it impossible to identify the health and use of services of such groups as young adults starting work, women of menopausal age, pre-retirement men.

2 The analyses for women by socio-economic group are never divided into those based on their husband's occupation and those based on their own.

3 Data about the specific conditions included in the check lists in 1977 and 1978 have not been presented.

4 In 1977 the analyses by illness and socio-economic group were not done by age. This makes them difficult to use and open to misuse since the proportion of men aged 65 or more rose from 7.5% in the professional group to 22.0% in the unskilled manual, while for women it rose from 6.2% to 35.6%. A footnote (on page 89 of the 1977 report) stating that 'the effect of standardisation would not be to eliminate any of the differences commented on, but only to reduce the variation slightly' leaves one in doubt about the differences presented but not discussed.

5 Data on use of services are rarely related to indicators of health.

This lack of published analyses would not matter so much if the data were readily accessible to other research workers. They are in fact deposited with the SSRC data bank, but the way the data have been processed has made them inaccessible to all but the most determined researchers with plenty of time to unravel the 'bewildering complexity' (Gilbert, Arber and Dale 1980).

This is one basic reason why this wealth of data has been underused. However, Gilbert, Arber and Dale have now converted the 1973–1976 GHS data into fully-labelled SPSS files and hope to complete the conversion of the 1977–1980 data by the end of 1983, so the data should be more accessible in the future, although there will still be a time lag.

Another handicap has been the inadequate staffing and time for analysis and writing at the Social Survey. As it stands the balance seems quite ludicrous – so much time and money is spent on collection of data, so little time and thought on their analysis. A third reason for the underuse of the data is the lack of validation.

Validation More experiments and validation exercises are needed to ascertain and demonstrate the usefulness and accuracy of the data. Some of these experiments need to be done separately from the GHS, for example among samples of patients whose responses could be compared with data from general practitioner records or with information from physical examinations. The sample sizes need not be large but some of the questions that need to be answered about existing data are:

1 How consistent are people in the way they report problems which are said to be recurring or present most of the time?
2 When people report such conditions as asthma, hay fever, blood pressure or heart trouble, has a doctor made such a diagnosis in the past and what diagnoses would doctors currently make?
3 When people are encouraged to think and talk about their health problems but are not presented with specific lists of conditions, how does the distribution of conditions they report compare with that obtained with the 1977–78 check lists?

Some comparisons and validations have been made in GHS reports. In 1972 GHS data on general practitioner consultations were compared with data from the national study of morbidity statistics from general practice. The two sets of consultation rates showed similar variations by age and sex but those from the general practitioners' records were markedly lower than those from the GHS. It was suggested that this was because the general practitioner study was based on volunteer, not random, practices. It would be useful to mount a study to find out how the accuracy with which patients report consultations compares with the accuracy with which doctors record them. It would be helpful if this could be answered for doctors in general and for doctors participating in the national studies of morbidity statistics from general practice. Without this sort of validation *Lancet* editorial writers may continue to press for the extension and strengthening of the national studies of morbidity statistics from general practice (*Lancet* 1981) without recognising that 'true morbidity data' are more likely to emanate from surveys such as the GHS.

The Nottingham health profile

This was developed as a result of 'a growing interest in sociomedical indicators which try to assess health in terms of "quality of life"' (Hunt et al 1980). In practice health is assessed negatively and it might more accurately be described as an illness profile. 'The Nottingham health profile is a two-part self-administered questionnaire . . . Part I consists of 38 statements with weighted scores in the areas of pain, physical mobility, sleep, energy, social isolation and emotional reactions' (Hunt, McKenna and Williams 1981). These are scored in such a way as to portray the severity of perceived dysfunction in the different domains. 'Part II is designed to give a general estimate of those areas of social function perceived to be affected by the health problems of the individual. This part contains a single statement on each of the following areas: paid employment, jobs around the home, social life, sex life, family relationships, hobbies/interests, and holidays.'

The profile was developed on the basis of interviews with patients with a variety of acute and chronic ailments. Scores from the questionnaires were related to medical information and independent assessments of patients' well-being (Hunt and McEwan 1980) and the seriousness weighted by using Thurstone's method of paired comparisons (McKenna, Hunt and McEwan 1981). It has been validated by demonstrating that it discriminates between groups differing in terms of diagnosed chronic illness, physiological fitness (Hunt et al 1980) and medical consultation (Hunt et al 1981).

Its reliability has been tested on patients with osteoarthritis who were given the questionnaire to fill in on two separate occasions four weeks apart (Hunt, McKenna and Williams 1981). Further tests of validity on different groups are planned. One rather disconcerting finding is that, contrary to logical expectation, there was no association between the number of respondents answering 'Yes' to an item and the perceived severity of that item. As the authors say 'this is an area for further investigation' (Hunt et al 1980).

Potentially this seems a useful tool. It has shown itself to be simple and short enough to be acceptable to elderly people. But the group who developed it has now largely dispersed and it remains to be seen whether it will be used by the individual members of the group or taken up by other workers.

In conclusion

A workshop was convened in 1978, with Sir John Brotherston in the chair: 'To assess what work could usefully be done to identify more direct indices of morbidity so that morbidity *per se* can be taken into account in the resource allocation process.' Forster (1978) reviewing various indicators of health care need considered the General Household Survey as the most suitable survey in this context, and showed that age standardised mortality in the ten regions of England and Wales did not correlate significantly with acute or bed sickness rates from the GHS but did so with its chronic sickness rates. Palmer (1978) pointed out that chronic sickness is more likely to include severe illnesses and disabilities. But the workshop concluded that the chief value of surveys was to deal with particular well-defined problems and only exceptionally could they be used to inform the more general process of decision making. Despite the limitations of the standardised mortality rate they concluded that this was for the present the best available indicator of morbidity and 'that it would be imprudent to replace it until a substantially better measure was available'.

In searching for general measures of health or sickness that can be ascertained by surveys and that can usefully and meaningfully be related to differences in services and to geographical, class and time variations, are we looking for an unobtainable philosopher's stone? I think there is some truth in this since surveys inevitably relate to people's perceptions about health and sickness and these are likely to differ between age, sex, socio-economic, educational, housing and geographical groups. But such differences can be illuminating in themselves and may stimulate the formulation of more precise theories. The measures are not particularly useful on their own, but only relatively. If we are to use them as indicators of need then we should show the way and the extent to which they are related to particular needs and in doing this we may find ways to sharpen the measures. But if we cannot define an ideal measure this should not deter us from making use of the practical tools that are available: we should concentrate on making these as useful and precise as we can. I think general indicators of health could usefully be obtained from the General Household Survey although I am critical of the ones that have been used up to now. At the same time I recognise the disadvantages of changing the questions yet again with the consequent loss of continuity.

One possibility that might be explored is including some questions on loss of function such as those asked in surveys of disability and discussed in a later chapter. An indication of the trends in the prevalence of disability and handicap could probably be obtained by asking relatively few questions. This seems a useful area to investigate since there may be an increasing prevalence of long-term disability in younger people as a result of a greater chance of survival of children born with abnormalities.

Another approach might be to include some or all of the questions from the Nottingham health profile. More validation exercises have been carried out on them than on the health questions in the GHS! But the GHS is the only national source of data on the health of people not using health services. In its way it takes the pulse of the nation at regular intervals. The potential is considerable; the achievement so far only modest.

3 *The nature of disease*

In this chapter I start by looking at a series of studies concerned to identify a factor related to disease. After that I review surveys aimed at the identification of a disease syndrome. Finally I describe the studies based on birth cohorts, which have illuminated the natural history of disease, its prevalence and its distribution.

Factors associated with disease

Studies in this field can have the excitement of the detective investigation: collecting evidence, identifying likely suspects, eliminating some suspects and pinpointing the villain. Unlike Sherlock Holmes's cases, in epidemiology there is seldom a single causal agent and there is never a confession. The challenge is to build up a watertight indictment by considering and eliminating alternative hypotheses. To illustrate the process I describe the classic studies on smoking and lung cancer by Doll and Hill (1950, 1952, 1954, 1956, 1964).

Their first study, published in 1950, was planned in 1947. At that time there had been a striking increase in lung cancer deaths during the preceding 25 years in this country and in others. One possibility was that this was due to improved standards of diagnosis, but Stocks (1947) pointed out that 'the increase of certified respiratory cancer mortality during the past 20 years has been as rapid . . . in country districts as in the cities with the best diagnostic facilities'. Doll and Hill state that two main causes had been put forward:

> '1. A general atmospheric pollution from the exhaust fumes of cars, from the surface dust of tarred roads and from gas works, industrial plants and coal fires.
> '2. The smoking of tobacco.'

They looked at the second possibility first, partly because there had been a number of small scale studies in which the smoking habits of lung cancer patients had been compared with other groups. Lung cancer patients appeared to be more likely to smoke at all and to smoke heavily.

Doll and Hill did the first part of their study in 20 London hospitals. The hospitals identified patients with cancer of the lung, stomach and large bowel – those with cancer of the stomach and large bowel being used for comparison. In addition they took a control group of non-cancer patients in the same hospitals matched with the lung cancer patients for sex and within the same five year age group. These patients were interviewed by almoners, working wholly on the study, who 'recorded the answers to a pre-arranged questionary' about their smoking habits.

One of the problems of this approach was that it was found impracticable for the interviewers to be unaware of the patient's diagnosis. This possible source of bias was discounted because there was a 'group of patients believed by the interviewers to have carcinoma of the lung at the time of interview, but who proved finally not to have that disease'. This group revealed a distribution of smoking habits similar to that shown by the other cancer and hospital patients but very different from that of the lung carcinoma patients.

Another point of concern was the reliability of the smoking histories that were reported. In an attempt to assess this, '50 unselected control patients with diseases other than cancer were interviewed a second time six months later'. A comparison of the results from the two interviews is given in Table 2. It shows good agreement.

Table 2 Amount of tobacco smoked daily before present illness as recorded at two interviews with the same patients at an interval of six months or more

First interview	Second interview						
	0	1 cig–	5 cigs–	15 cigs–	25 cigs–	50 cigs–	Total
0	8	1					9
1 cig–		4	1				5
5 cigs–		1	13	3			17
15 cigs–			4	9	1		14
25 cigs–				1	3	—	4
50 cigs–					1	—	1
Total	8	6	18	13	5	—	50

A third source of anxiety was the control group which had been matched for sex and five year age group with the lung cancer patients. The social class distributions of the patients and controls were similar but places of residence showed a large difference. This was thought to be because lung cancer patients came to specialist hospitals from a wider area. When the comparison was confined to patients seen at district (non-specialist) hospitals in London the difference disappeared.

Another survey of the general population was used to check the possibility that the control group were for any reason particularly light smokers. The comparison was made after standardisation for age and showed that somewhat heavier smoking habits had been recorded among the patients with diseases other than lung cancer than in the sample of the general public.

In discussing the data from their preliminary report, Doll and Hill concluded that there is a real association between carcinoma of the lung and smoking, but pointed out that this was not necessarily to say that smoking causes carcinoma of the lung. 'The association would occur if carcinoma of the lung caused people to smoke or if both attributes were end-effects of a common cause.' They went on to point out: '. . . the habit of smoking was . . . invariably formed before the onset of the disease . . . so that the disease cannot be held to have caused the habit'.

Between January 1950 and February 1952 they extended their study to hospitals in Bristol, Cambridge, Leeds and Newcastle and also further patients from eight of the initial 20 London hospitals. This time the hospitals were asked to identify only patients with carcinoma of the lung and the matched control patients included, with certain exceptions, other forms of cancer. In their 1952 report they also considered other aetiological factors, including place of residence, residence near a gasworks, use of petrol lighters, exposure to different forms of heating and previous respiratory illness.

The nature of the sample is not ideal for considering differences between town and country because of the possibly different areas from which lung cancer patients and others were likely to be drawn. But they found that in the provinces a smaller proportion of the lung carcinoma than the control patients lived in the country and concluded that this supported the contention that lung carcinoma is less common in rural than in urban areas.

They also discussed the suggestion that subjects with a particular physical constitution might be prone to develop the habit of smoking and lung cancer but stated that they knew of no evidence of such a relationship. Another possibility discussed was a relationship between the development of lung cancer and an attack of influenza during the pandemic of 1918–19. But they put forward evidence from other countries and of the similar incidence of influenza in men and women which made such a theory seem implausible.

They used the study data to make estimates of the risk of smoking different amounts and types (cigarettes or pipe) of tobacco, and they looked at inhaling, the use of cigarette holders and at filter-tipped or other cigarettes.

Their conclusion from both the preliminary and the later study was that the association between carcinoma of the lung and smoking was real. Their caveats to the later, 1952, report were rather different from those to the earlier one: 'It is not argued that tobacco smoke contributes to the development of all cases of the disease – a most unlikely event. It is not argued that it is the sole cause of the increased death rate of recent years nor that it can wholly explain the different mortality rates between town and country.'

A leader in the *British Medical Journal* (1952) was more outspoken. 'Where do we go from here? Statistics, it is said, cannot prove causation . . . All that these things can do is to show that the probability of a causative connection between an agent and a disease is so great that we are bound to take what preventive action we can, accepting the theory as though the proof were absolute until further research leads to some modification. It would seem that such a position has now been reached with lung carcinoma, in that tobacco has now been incriminated as the vehicle conveying an agent responsible for a large proportion of the cases. The nature of the carcinogenic agent is not yet known.' Johnston (1952) went further, describing Doll and Hill's second article as 'a most comprehensive and satisfying account . . . [it] confirms and greatly strengthens their previous conclusion that smoking is an important factor in the production of cancer of the lung. They have again refrained, however, from suggesting a specific measure, (or measures) to be taken appropriate to their findings. . . . Both the investigators and the writer of your leading article have lacked the guts to state the obvious and only rational conclusion to be drawn from these findings – that tobacco smoking should be prevented completely, and as soon as possible.'

However the Minister of Health, Mr Iain Macleod, although he stated in Parliament: '. . . it must be regarded as established that there is a relationship between smoking and cancer of the lung' considered that the time had not yet come when the Ministry should issue public warnings against smoking; this, although he acknowledged 'a strong presumption that the relationship is causal'. His reservations apparently arose because the presence in tobacco of a carcinogenic agent causing lung cancer was not yet certain; there was evidence that the increase in lung cancer over time was not entirely due to smoking;

and it appeared that atmospheric pollution and occupational hazards might be contributing to lung cancer (*British Medical Journal 1954*).

Doll and Hill sought further evidence. In 1954, after quoting still further studies of the association between tobacco smoking and lung cancer they said: 'Some have considered that the only reasonable explanation is that smoking is a factor in the production of the disease: others have not been prepared to deduce causation and have left the association unexplained. . . . Further retrospective studies of that same kind would seem to us unlikely to advance our knowledge materially or to throw any new light upon the nature of the association. If too, there were any undetected flaws in the evidence that such studies have produced it would be exposed only by some entirely new approach. That approach we considered should be "prospective".'

For this prospective study they decided to study British doctors, sending postal questionnaires in 1951 to the 59,600 men and women on the current British Medical Register. The questionnaires were about smoking habits and they estimated that they obtained replies from 69% of the men and 60% of the women who were alive at the time of the inquiry. Through the Registrar Generals they obtained information about the cause of death registered for every doctor after the questionnaires were sent out.

As they expected death rates were relatively low among responders initially since the seriously ill would have been unable or reluctant to reply. In their preliminary 1954 report they found 'a significant and steadily rising mortality from deaths due to cancer of the lung as the amount of tobacco smoked increases'. In a second report on the study in 1956, with a considerably increased body of data, these findings were confirmed. In addition they were able to look at doctors who had given up smoking at the time of their inquiry in 1951. A comparison between them and those who reported themselves as smokers revealed a progressive and significant reduction in mortality with the increase in the length of time over which smoking had been given up.

In 1957 the Medical Research Council issued a statement on tobacco smoking and lung cancer. Its conclusions were:

'1. A very great increase has occurred during the past 25 years in the death rate from lung cancer in Great Britain and other countries.

'2. A relatively small number of the total cases can be attributed to specific industrial hazards.

'3. A proportion of cases, the exact extent of which cannot yet be defined, may be due to atmospheric pollution.

'4. Evidence from many investigations in different countries indicates that a major part of the increase is associated with tobacco smoking, particularly in the form of cigarettes. In the opinion of the Council, the most reasonable interpretation of this evidence is that the relationship is one of direct cause and effect.

'5. The identification of several carcinogenic substances in tobacco smoke provides a rational basis for such a causal relationship.'

A leader in the *British Medical Journal* (1957) discussed this statement. It refers to 'the painstaking investigations of statisticians that seem to have closed every loophole of escape for tobacco as the villain in the piece' and says that 'it is as well to remember that now for a great many years clinicians have been convinced of a causal connexion between cigarette smoking and lung cancer'. The same leader also reported that the Imperial Tobacco Company had set up the Tobacco Manufacturers Standing Committee 'to assist research into smoking and health questions . . . and to make information available to scientific workers and the public'. Sir Ronald Fisher had agreed to be one of its scientific consultants.

The next issue of the *British Medical Journal* contained a letter from R A Fisher (1957a). In it he described the contention that painstaking investigations . . . have closed every loophole of escape for tobacco as the villain as 'pure political rhetoric' and referred to, but did not identify, 'alternative explanation of the facts which still await exclusion'.

A month later Fisher (1957b) was more explicit, and discussed 'two classes of alternative theories which any statistical association, observed without the precautions of a definite experiment, always allows – namely 1) that the supposed effect is really the cause, or in this case that incipient cancer, or a precancerous condition with chronic inflammation, is a factor in inducing the smoking of cigarettes, or 2) that cigarette smoking and lung cancer, though not mutually causative are both influenced by a common cause, in this case the individual genotype'. He went on to say that 'the belief that cigarette smoking causes lung cancer would be more secure if [it was] not encumber[ed] with the non sequitur that increase of smoking is the cause of increasing cancer of the lung'. He further argued: 'When the sexes are compared it is found that lung cancer has been increasing more rapidly in men relatively to women. The absolute rate of increase is, of course, obscured by improved methods of diagnosis, and by the increased attention paid to the disease, but the relative proportionate changes in men and women should be free from these disturbances, and the change has gone decidedly against the men. But it is notorious, and conspicuous in the memory of most of us, that over the last 50 years the increase of smoking among women has been great, and that among men (even if positive) certainly small. The theory that increased smoking is "the cause" of the change in apparent incidence of lung cancer is not even tenable in face of this contrast.' He concluded: '. . . it will be as clear in retrospect, as it is now in logic, that the data so far do not warrant the conclusions based on them'.

In the following year, writing in *Nature*, Fisher (1958a) presented some results of an inquiry into the smoking habits of adult male twin pairs in support of his argument about genetic links. Among the 51 monozygotic pairs, 33 were 'wholly alike qualitatively' while among the 31 dizygotics 'only eleven can be classed as wholly alike'.

In a subsequent letter (1958b) presenting further data of this sort, this time relating to female twins, he also refers to data about inhaling and lung cancer and concludes: 'There is nothing to stop those who greatly desire it from believing that lung cancer is caused by smoking cigarettes. They should also believe that inhaling cigarette smoke is a protection. To believe either is, however, to run the risk of failing to recognize, and therefore failing to prevent, other and more genuine causes.'

Doll and Hill did not enter into this correspondence. They persisted with their studies, sending a second questionnaire to male doctors in 1957–58 and to female doctors in 1960–61. This covered their smoking history since the earlier study. In 1964 they reported that after ten years the death rates for men were high among smokers for '. . . cancer of the lung, cancer of the upper respiratory and digestive tracts, chronic bronchitis, pulmonary tuberculosis, coronary disease without hypertension, peptic ulcer, cirrhosis of the liver and alcoholism. No association was found with the remaining 61% of the death rate . . . In men who have given up cigarette smoking the death rate from cancer of lung falls substantially. It continues to fall step by step the longer smoking has been given up. This trend can be explained in terms of a diminishing risk from the previously operative environmental agent, but not in terms of genetic selection of those who choose to give up.'

A leader in the *British Medical Journal* (1964) commented: 'The most important practical conclusion that must be drawn from the study is that cigarette smoking now kills thousands of men and women every year.' And in a letter to the *Journal* Sir Cecil Wakeley, Chairman of the Council of the Imperial Cancer Research Fund, who had been quoted in a *British Medical Journal* leader as saying 'smoking 10 to 15 cigarettes a day is no more likely to give you cancer than if you did not smoke at all', conceded: 'I recognise that although the development of bronchial carcinoma is materially less in light smokers than in heavy smokers the evidence available shows that smoking cigarettes, even in small numbers, adds to the hazard in comparison with non smokers. I would like therefore to make it clear that the views of the Imperial Cancer Research Fund on this subject do not differ from those expressed in the reports of the Medical Research Council, the Royal College of Physicians and the Surgeon General of the United States, which have been reinforced more recently by the latest publications of Dr Richard Doll and Sir Austin Bradford Hill.'

The story illustrates the limits of the usefulness of surveys in a number of ways. First, the initial hypothesis that smoking causes lung cancer did not result from survey data but from clinical observation. Second, association does not imply causation: other explanations need to be examined and excluded before causation should be assumed, and even then some logical, and possibly many political, economic and emotional reservations remain. Third, there is the importance of the relationship between survey and other data – in this instance laboratory studies and experimental work. The likely implication from the survey data that smoking caused lung cancer became more plausible and acceptable once it had been shown that tobacco contained carcinogenic agents. Finally, and related to the other points, are the factors which influence the acceptability of evidence from surveys. It seems that smoking would have been more readily accepted as a cause of lung cancer if it had been the only cause, and if the association had explained all the other variations in the incidence of lung cancer. In addition it is likely that it would have been more readily accepted if it had not had such obvious economic implications for the tobacco industry and also, in terms of tax revenue, for the Treasury.

Identification of disease syndromes

Another concern of epidemiology is the identification of syndromes, since the pattern and associations of symptoms and signs contribute to the identification and understanding of disease. (For a discussion about this see Morris 1957). Surveys are of use in this field too and the example I have taken here is the menopausal syndrome. The basic questions are: does it exist and if so what symptoms are associated with it? In an attempt to answer these, Thompson, Hart and Durno (1973) sent a questionnaire to all the women aged between 40 and 60 years in a practice in Aberdeen asking about menstrual history, twelve different symptoms and various demographic details. The response rate was 92%. Results were analysed separately for those who had an artificial menopause (as a result of surgical intervention) and those experiencing, or at risk to, a natural one. The conclusion was that as far as symptoms were concerned, only the vasomotor disorders, flushing and night sweats, were definitely correlated with the menopause. McKinlay and Jefferys (1974) and McKinlay, Jefferys and Thompson (1972) had carried out a somewhat similar study on a larger sample from eight practices in or near London. They got an 82% response to a postal questionnaire sent to 955 women aged 45–54. The eight symptoms they asked about were hot flushes, night sweats, headaches, dizzy spells, palpitations, sleeplessness, depression and weight increase. They too found that hot flushes and night sweats were clearly associated with the onset of a natural menopause but the other six symptoms showed no direct relationship with it.

Bungay, Vessey and McPherson (1980) criticised both these studies, and others, on the grounds that they were discernible as being concerned with the menopause, 'thereby almost certainly introducing bias into the responses'. Their study incorporated three 'special features . . . in an attempt to improve on earlier work'. First they surveyed men as well as women, 'the men in a sense serving as controls'; second they covered a broad age band, 30–64 years; and third they used two postal questionnaires, despatched with an interval of six to eight weeks. The first questionnaire inquired about 40 symptoms relating to various physical, sexual and emotional problems; no mention was made of the menopause either in the questionnaire or the covering letter which stated that the study was concerned with the health problems of men and women of working age. The second questionnaire, which was sent only to people responding to the first one, was concerned with family, social, gynaecological and treatment matters which they felt might have biased responses to the first if they had not been separated. The response rate for the pair of questionnaires was 72% for women and 68% for men – lower than either of the other two studies. However, using two separate questionnaires did not reduce it by much, as 94% of the second questionnaires were completed.

They analysed their data by sex and five-year age groups and interpreted the resulting symptom curves by 'visual recognition of patterns'. They identified three basic hypothetical types: the first with parallel male and female curves, the second with male and female curves not parallel but with the female pattern not related to the mean age at menopause, and the third with male and female curves not parallel and the female pattern related to mean age at menopause. Examination of the data led them to subdivide the third type into symptoms whose prevalence for women peaked around the mean age of menopause (type 3a) and those for which the 'curve for women changed direction, starting around the time of menopause' (type 3b).

In their paper they presented graphical data for four symptoms with type 3a patterns: flushing, sweating by night, difficulty making decisions and loss of confidence, and stated that 'the peaks of prevalence of night sweats, day sweats and flushing in women are clearly associated with the mean age of menopause'. They also noted that: 'The less impressive peaks of prevalence of a group of mental symptoms (difficulty with decisions and concentration, anxiety, loss of confidence, feelings of unworthiness and forgetfulness) are clearly associated with an age just preceding the mean age of menopause. This holds also for the small peaks for dizziness, tiredness and palpitations'. Results for three symptoms identified as being of type 3b are presented in graphical form, along with the statement: 'The type 3b patterns for aching breasts and irritability suggest that these symptoms are associated with the menstrual cycle and diminish after the menopause. The explanation of the similar pattern of low backache in women is less obvious.'

Bungay and his colleagues attempted to analyse the data by menopause state and chronological age but reported that large numbers would be needed to obtain clear results. They concluded: '. . . the data suggested, however, that vasomotor symptoms are more closely related to menopausal state, and mental symptoms to chronological age'.

Symptom patterns by age and sex, showing different types of responses

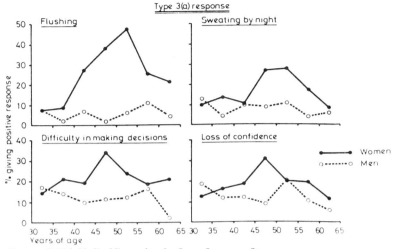

Source: British Medical Journal, vol. 281, 1980, page 182

In addition, they collected data about such 'life events' as the death of a close relative, serious illness in the family and unemployment and found little evidence that such problems clustered around the mean age of menopause. 'More women in their forties and fifties, however, reported that their children were leaving home, marrying, or causing special worry than did younger or older women. These events were positively associated with the reporting of symptoms, but the distinctive patterns already described were clearly apparent in women who claimed that they had no problems with their children.' They did not present data about these analyses for the men in their sample.

Thompson and her colleagues and McKinlay and hers both identified the vasomotor disorders as the only definite symptoms associated with the menopause. And while Bungay et al supported this, 'our study supports the view that there is a menopausal syndrome (principally affecting vasomotor symptoms)', their data also showed peaks of prevalence around the menopause for a number of mental symptoms. The number of women covered in their study was of a similar order to that studied by McKinlay et al, so that cannot account for the difference between the significances of the results which might have been expected to be in the opposite direction, with Bungay et al showing fewer associations, if the bias had existed. The graphical presentations of Bungay and his colleagues make it difficult to quote their data or check the significance of their results. And they stated that they 'interpreted the symptom curves by visual recognition of patterns rather than by any formal statistical approach'. In addition they presented only a selection of even their positive findings. While they maintained that vasomotor symptoms are more closely related to menopausal state, and mental symptoms to chronological age, the picture for the two mental symptoms presented suggest that their effect is more transitory – a somewhat surprising finding.

Another problem with the data from Bungay et al is that they related their findings simply to average age at menopause and they did not define this in their paper. McKinlay and her colleagues on the other hand distinguished three categories of menopausal status in their main analyses: 1 premenopausal – menstruated within the last three months; 2 menopausal – last menstruated between three and 12 months ago; 3 postmenopausal – not menstruated within the last 12 months.

So while the study design of Bungay et al was innovative and imaginative, the classification, analysis and presentation of the results seem less satisfactory. And no further data have been published from the study. It has removed any remaining doubts about one aspect of the menopausal syndrome but it would seem that the association of mental symptoms with the menopausal syndrome is still in doubt. As Bungay and his colleagues point out, all the studies, including theirs, have been carried out at one point in time but the data have been interpreted longitudinally. In theory some of the associations could be attributable to differences between successive cohorts, though this seems unlikely. They regard a follow-up study tracing an individual group of women throughout middle life as extremely difficult to conduct and demanding great resources. However the first national birth cohort of 1946 will pass through the menopause before the end of the century; possibly their experience will be documented. This would seem a more satisfactory approach since the menopause is a phase that can only be identified in retrospect.

The birth cohort studies

In Britain there have been three national cohort studies based on births, or notifications of births, during one week in 1946, 1958 and 1970. In the first study, which came to be known as the National

Survey of Health and Development, it was hoped to interview all women delivered in England, Scotland and Wales during the week 3–9 March 1946. There were some initial losses, amounting to about 8%, because some local authorities refused to cooperate and a further 2% were lost because of late notification. Among the remaining 15,130, 90.5% were successfully interviewed by health visitors about eight weeks after the birth. The main emphasis of this part of the study was on the social and economic aspects of pregnancy and childbirth (Douglas 1948).

From this sample of 13,687 births, 5,362 children were selected for follow-up. Twins and illegitimate births were excluded and the sample was deliberately weighted in order to get roughly equal numbers of manual and non-manual workers' children. Contacts with the children were made at intervals of two years or less until they were 26 years old, and after that at intervals of five years or less up to 36 years so far. Their children are now being followed up. These contacts were made by a variety of people: health visitors, school nurses, school doctors, school teachers, youth employment officers and professional interviewers. Because the sample is scattered without any clustering over the whole country, considerable organisation was involved. It meant that it was expensive to use professional interviewers as they had to travel long distances, so locally based health professionals collected most of the data during the childhood of the cohort. This had some advantages and some disadvantages: professionals could make professional assessments but they lacked research interviewing skills and, because of their professional involvement, they might elicit biased responses to some questions. In addition they had to complete the study records on top of their usual activities. Postal questionnaires were not used until after the children had left school and only ocasionally since because it was felt important to have personal contact and to establish involvement in the project. The success of this strategy was illustrated by the fact that 25 years after the start of the project approximately 4,500 were known to be still living in Great Britain and contact was made with 4,041 of them. (Douglas, Kiernan and Wadsworth 1977).

Later interests in the study were on education (Douglas 1964, Douglas, Ross and Simpson 1968) and delinquency (Wadsworth 1979). But the study was also concerned with the natural history of disease and with medical policies and their effects. Some of the epidemiological issues which the study illuminated were social class differences in health and survival during the first two years of life (Douglas 1951), the development of premature children (Douglas and Mogford 1953a and 1963b, Douglas 1956a and 1956b), the prevalence of bedwetting (Blomfield and Douglas 1956), air pollution and respiratory illness in childhood (Douglas and Waller 1966); chronic illness in childhood (Pless and Douglas 1971), respiratory disease in young adults (Colley, Douglas and Reid 1973), the relationship between age at puberty and age at marriage and first parenthood (Kiernan 1977), the long-term effects of breast feeding (Marmot, Page, Atkins and Douglas 1980) and a longitudinal study of obesity (Stark, Atkins, Wolff and Douglas 1981).

The focus of the 1958 birth cohort study was initially on perinatal mortality (Butler and Bonham 1963, Butler and Alberman 1969). Again the main sample was confined to a single week but perinatal deaths in a longer period were included; these were examined by pathologists and their findings recorded on standardised forms. On this cohort the children were followed up when they were seven (Pringle, Butler and Davie 1966 and Davie, Butler and Goldstein 1972), eleven (Davie 1973) and sixteen (Fogelman 1976). Many of the reports from this study have focused on particular groups: the adopted, the illegitimate, those in one-parent families or in care, those with speech defects, hearing loss, diabetes and epilepsy. And issues related to education, housing, poverty and the family received more attention than health and handicap.

Both the 1946 and 1958 cohort studies have been, and still are, a goldmine for data in such a wide variety of fields that it seems inappropriate to focus on particular aspects.

The British Births Survey, 1970, covered all babies born alive or dead after the 24th week of gestation (not the 28th as in the 1958 study) during the week beginning 5 April 1970. Reports have been published on the first week of life (Chamberlain et al 1975) and on obstetric care (Chamberlain et al 1978). Two follow-up studies of the whole cohort have been carried out when the children were five and ten years old.

The possibility of carrying out a fourth cohort study based on births in 1982 was considered by the National Perinatal Epidemiology Unit but after much discussion and consultation it was decided not to do so. One problem with such a series is that each one seems to involve wider professional involvement and consultation. The initial 1946 study was undertaken by a joint committee of the Royal College of Obstetricians and Gynaecologists and the Population Investigation Committee. The committee had a chairman, secretary, eleven members, a director (J W B Douglas) and a research assistant. The first book on the study, *Maternity in Great Britain*, was published in 1948, two years later. The 1958 study was done under the auspices of the National Birthday Trust Fund. The steering committee had a chairman, sixteen members plus fourteen nominated representatives from various organisations and eight observers from government departments and the Central Midwives Board. There was also a pathology sub-committee with nine members. The first report on the study, *Perinatal Mortality*, was published five years after the study was carried out. The steering committee for the 1970 study had a chairman, fourteen members, 29 nominated representatives, fourteen observers, an initial working party with ten members, four working parties on the content of the survey (obstetric, paediatric, socio-economic and medical care administration) another working party on the final arrangements for the survey, and in addition six members of the Scientific Advisory Committee for the National Birthday Trust Fund attending meetings as did four other people by invitation. The first report again appeared five years later.

Proposals for a fourth national perinatal study (Golding 1979) were elaborate and ambitious. They included a prospective element, the suggestion being that all women reporting themselves as pregnant during a relatively long period of time should keep, in booklet form, records of various aspects of their pregnancy, with details of hospital admissions, medicine taking, symptoms, work, smoking, alcohol consumption, weight, and so on. This was in addition to the 'traditional sample' of births in a particular period and additional samples of still births, neonatal deaths and a further sample of low birthweight live births. Reasons for rejecting the proposals reflect a disenchantment with the approach – the 1970 study had been something of a disappointment and had not made a major impact on practice. In addition the estimated costs of the new study were felt to be high. Other reasons were that previous surveys had yielded few insights about aetiological agents of perinatal mortality and morbidity – with the notable exception of the relationship between maternal smoking and adverse outcome of pregnancy (Fedrick, Alberman and Goldstein 1971, Butler, Goldstein and Ross 1972).

The outstanding achievements of the birth cohort studies have been to provide a basis for longitudinal studies and a variety of representative samples of children with particular problems. One disadvantage of the 1946 cohort is that the sample became less representative as the children grew older since there were no attempts, for instance, to identify immigrants who were born during the study weeks. But this has been done on the other two cohorts. Another problem is the seasonal bias for conditions with the month of birth or conception. This last difficulty could have been overcome if births had been sampled throughout a year. Douglas himself has said (1976): 'If I were to repeat the 1946 study I would take a six-day sample spread throughout the year.' If other methods of sample selection had been used it would have been possible to cluster births geographically so that it would have been more feasible, because less expensive, to use professional interviewers rather than health visitors, midwives and teachers to collect some of the information.

One possible snag in these longitudinal studies is the possible effect of the study on the children who are followed up so frequently. Douglas (1976) was able to make one check on this effect by comparing the 'rejects' from the 1946 cohort with those who were included in it when they were eleven years old. Both groups were examined by a school doctor and their mothers were interviewed. Minor speech and eye defects had more often been treated among those included in the longitudinal study, but there was no evidence of a major bias. But as Douglas pointed out 'we have no assurance that biases are absent in the middle-class group of children for whom we have no controls'.

In theory, the existence of three cohort studies at twelve year intervals is a tremendous opportunity to study changes over time and the effects of different policies and practices. But this has been exploited very little – apart from comparisons of tonsillectomy and circumcision between two cohorts (Calnan, Douglas and Goldstein 1978). One reason for the lack of comparison is that few data were recorded or questions asked and recorded in a strictly comparable way. Because of this considerable opportunities were lost.

Methodological issues

The various methodological issues which have been illustrated by the studies discussed in this chapter relate to study design, validation, response rates, analysis, presentation and acceptance.

Study design In the surveys of the menopause, the design of Bungay and his colleagues, with the data collected by two separate questionnaires, elegantly avoids the possible bias of contamination. The results suggest that the bias did not exist in practice – although it was useful to demonstrate this.

The first birth cohort study became less representative of the population as the children grew older. But on the later cohorts immigrants born during the study week were identified and included.

The studies of lung cancer and smoking confronted a number of design problems. There was the difficulty of obtaining appropriate controls. Taking other hospital patients created problems in pin-pointing urban/rural differences between the two groups. But it is difficult to identify any appropriate alternatives. At that time few general practitioners had age-sex registers so they were not a practical source. The initial use of a retrospective design produced results relatively quickly and their findings were strengthened by being supported by results from a subsequent prospective study. Using doctors for the prospective study had a number of advantages: a list, likely to be relatively complete, was readily available; doctors were comparatively unlikely to change their occupation; their occupation was likely to be recorded reasonably accurately on the death certificate; and the majority were men. An additional advantage emerged during the course of the study: a relatively high proportion of them gave up smoking which enabled Doll and Hill to assess the effects of this.

Validation One problem of Doll and Hill's design was that the interviewing could not be done 'blind' – the interviewers were often aware of the patient's diagnosis. Doll and Hill opportunistically made use of a group of patients who turned out to have been initially misdiagnosed to show that the lack of blindness was unlikely to have biased the findings. They also arranged for some of the controls to be re-interviewed in order to assess the reliability of the reported smoking histories, and demonstrated that the accounts were at any rate mainly repeatable.

Another way of validating survey data was adopted by Douglas on the first birth cohort study. His concern was to assess the effects of the series of surveys on the children involved and to show that the study had not influenced behaviour and attitudes. He did this by a single follow up of those who had been excluded from the cohort.

Response rates were generally good on the cohort studies and on those concerned with the menopause syndrome. In Doll and Hill's 1952 study none of the 3,208 patients refused to be interviewed, but

15% were not seen because they had already been discharged from hospital, were too ill, or had died. That no patients refused is, in my view, a cause of some concern suggesting that patients may have felt unable to do so. Response rates to the postal questionnaires to doctors were surprisingly low: 69% for the men, 60% for the women; possibly they omitted to send the usual two reminders.

Analysis One problem of commission and one of omission were identified. The commission relates to the use of the average age at menopause that Bungay and his colleagues used to interpret their data. The omission seems much more important and concerns the almost complete lack of comparison between the three birth cohort studies. Part of the 'explanation' seems to lie in the way the data were obtained and classified, but whatever the reason valuable opportunities have been missed.

Presentation The graphical presentation adopted by Bungay and his colleagues restricts the amount of data presented, inhibits precise quotation and comparison of their findings and makes it impossible to check the significance of their results.

On the lung cancer and smoking studies, when Doll and Hill presented their findings did they cling too rigidly to the strictly scientific limitations of their data? By not being prepared to say, at an earlier stage, that on the basis of their evidence they believed that the only reasonable interpretation was that smoking caused lung cancer did they delay the time at which the Government was prepared to take any stance or action? Did they put strict scientific standards above humanitarian considerations? If so, were they right to do so? I am uncertain.

4 Assessment of needs

Chapter 2 was concerned with general measures of health and sickness which might be taken as broad, non-specific indicators of need. This one is about surveys of the needs of particular groups. It starts with two groups which are likely to have a wide variety of needs: the handicapped or disabled and the dying; and then looks at studies of two groups with specific problems: those with incontinence and those having trouble with their feet. The chapter starts with a discussion of what is meant by need.

The definition of need

Bradshaw (1972) identified four types of need, which he described as normative, felt need or want, expressed need and comparative need. The first is that which the expert or professional defines as need in any given situation: its definition may change in time as a result of developments in knowledge, the changing values of society or the value orientation of the expert. Felt need, or want, is related to the perceptions of the individual. Expressed need or demand is felt need turned into action. A measure of comparative need is obtained by studying the characteristics of the population in receipt of a service and defining those with similar characteristics as in need. This chapter is mainly concerned with the first two types, need defined by the expert and felt need, and the last one, comparative need. The next chapter, which is about the use of services, relates to expressed need and also discusses comparative need.

Studies of the handicapped and disabled

The basic questions posed in these surveys were first how many people were handicapped and disabled, and then what sort of needs did they have? Before discussing the studies it is helpful to define the various concepts that are used in terms of the most recent World Health Organization classification (1980). This defines *impairment* as any loss or abnormality of psychological, physiological or anatomical structure or function; *disability* as any restriction or lack of ability (resulting from an impairment) to perform an activity in the manner or within the range considered normal for a human being; and *handicap* as the disadvantage resulting from impairment or disability.

A study carried out by OPCS before these terms had been defined in precisely these ways but adopting a similar although somewhat narrower perspective was '. . . designed to give reliable estimates of the number of handicapped people aged 16 and over, living in private households in Great Britain' (Harris 1971). It was done in two stages. At the first stage, a postal questionnaire was sent to a random sample of just under 250,000 addresses asking about various impairments and about such things as difficulty in going up or down stairs, or in gripping or holding things, experienced by any of the adults (aged 16 or over) living in the study households. Replies were received from 86%. The possibility that the impaired would be more likely to respond to the study was considered; but the proportion impaired was similar among those responding at different intervals so it was assumed that non-respondents did not differ significantly from the respondents in whether or not they were impaired. The postal inquiry was designed to identify two samples. The first was concerned with people with any disability and in this sample all positive responses relating to people aged under 65 were followed up by interview and one in four of those relating to people aged 65 or more. The second sample was concerned with the very severely handicapped and those needing special care, but of those identified in the postal screen over half, 58%, proved ineligible. While the postal screen identified many false positives there was apparently no check on possible false negatives. In a local study in Canterbury, Warren (1975) attempted to do this by a search of the records of 15 agencies. He found that 65% of those on the agency records had been identified as handicapped or impaired in the household survey while 36% of all those so identified in the household survey were on the records of the agencies. Further analysis found 'no evidence to suggest that the short fall of the household survey was greater than 10%'. Returning to Harris's study, 89% of the eligibles in the first sample and 85% of those in the second were successfully interviewed. The interview schedule for the first sample has been described by Alderson and Dowie (1979, page 82) as 'a tremendous document, with 150 questions'. In addition some tests of motor capacity were carried out. A functional classification of handicap was developed, based on the amount of help individuals required in daily self-care. This classification was based on replies to questions and not on performance of the tests. A subsequent analysis of the relationship between the performance of the tests and the categories of self-care found that the two measures corresponded relatively closely (Jefferys et al 1969). One problem was that the tests were often not acceptable to the very old or severely handicapped living in their own homes.

The methods and scope of the OPCS study reflect a concern for what was regarded as 'hard' precise data. Physical tests were applied and the questions related to activities and the physical environment. Contacts with others were viewed in the context of the person's ability to reach desired destinations and whether he or she had a telephone. A wide range of possible aids to handicap were considered, from automobiles and attendance at clubs to walking sticks and washing machines. But the questions mainly covered the help the handicapped got and the things they had difficulty in doing or could not do, and only a few asked directly about perceptions of unmet need. The needs identified in this study were mainly normative, the criteria being laid down, or left to, the professionals.

Following this survey many local authorities carried out somewhat similar inquiries to ascertain the prevalence of impairment and handicap in their areas. (See Knight and Warren 1978, for a description of the studies and a critique of their methods and results). A number of these studies aimed at identifying disabled people in order to help them directly, so they covered the total population not just a sample. Being based on the OPCS model (Harris and Head 1971 and 1974) these studies too were mainly concerned with normative and comparative needs. Some 'felt that a direct question on need would be inappropriate if the need could not be met, and preferred to estimate need from a person's handicap and home support' (Knight and Warren 1978, page 50).

More recently a study based on the wider concepts of handicap and disability in the 1980 WHO definition has been carried out in Lambeth in 1978 (Patrick et al 1981). This included 25 screening items on disability covering mobility, body care and movement, sensory-motor dysfunction and limitation of social activity. Eleven of the 25 were items covered in the national OPCS study (Harris 1971) so comparisons could be made between the two. These showed that in relation to the eleven items the overall prevalence rate, relating to the number of people with one or more impairment or disability, was 7.9% in the 1978 Lambeth study and 7.8% in the 1968/69 national one. But with the 25 items the estimated prevalence rate for Lambeth was 15.4%. 'Sensory-motor items such as frequent falls, and occupation related items such as difficulty doing job of choice or housework, significantly increase reported disability.'

So, as with surveys of general measures of health or sickness, the amount, level and nature of disability revealed varies greatly and depends on the questions asked. The results from the 1978 Lambeth survey were also compared with an earlier one, 1966–7, in the same area (Bennett, Garrad and Halil 1970). Analysis of the responses to specific items indicated the effect of question wording in that the 1968 study included questions on people's *capacity* or ability to perform certain activity while the 1978 survey asked what they did – that is, their *performance*. Patrick and his colleagues concluded: '. . . as performance is more readily observable and objective than capacity the questions on capacity might well be abandoned for measures of self reported disability'.

Another methodological observation from the study by Patrick and his colleagues was that a significantly higher proportion of the disabled than the non-disabled were identified during the earlier postal phase of the study compared with the later phase when non-respondents were followed up with home visits by medical students. This contrasts with the finding of Harris (1971).

The studies of Harris and of Patrick and his colleagues related disability to the conditions which caused it. This illuminates needs for certain types of medical services and, importantly, Warren (1976) has shown that reliable data about the nature of conditions causing disability can be obtained in interview studies. He checked 311 statements by impaired people and reported that 94% were corroborated by the general practitioner, and that the survey data was more likely to be deficient rather than inaccurate in relation to specific diseases and especially in relation to causes of deafness, sight difficulties and musculoskeletal disorders.

Alongside the Lambeth health survey of Patrick and his colleagues there is also '*a study of the social and economic consequences of disability* to develop an understanding of handicap and how it is influenced by the social situations of physically impaired and disabled persons and a *priorities study* to examine the preference for cash benefits *or* local authority services held by disabled people, the relatives and friends who care for them, and the planners and providers of these services' (Patrick 1981).

In a related study Patrick, Peach and Gregg (1982) designed an inquiry to assess general practitioners' knowledge of their disabled patients. It was carried out in one, six-doctor practice. They found that the general practitioners 'knew of only 50% of the difficulties with daily living reported by the disabled and even less of the aids, appliances and services used'.

In the same exercise this group also compared results from postal and interviewer administered questionnaires for identifying disabled persons (Peach, Green, Locker, Darby and Patrick 1980). They did this by interviewing people who had completed a postal questionnaire and found that the interviewer-administered questionnaire produced fewer positive responses to a list of problems than the postal one. But in their published report they only compared the distributions and presented no cross analyses, so have not demonstrated the repeatability of individual items. However Peach (personal communication) has carried out such analyses and found that congruity was high. He and his colleagues concluded that the postal questionnaire was a reliable instrument for identifying the disabled since none of their sample was classified differently as disabled or non-disabled by the two methods. However their sample of 25 non-disabled people seems unusual as none of them had seen their general practitioner within the twelve months preceding or succeeding the date on which they were interviewed. Less than a fifth of the general population of adults is estimated to fall into this group (Cartwright and Anderson 1981 additional unpublished data). I think Peach and his colleagues have demonstrated that postal surveys are certainly superior to general practitioner records and recollections in identifying the disabled; but the relative reliability of the postal study and interview survey seem less well established from their data.

Neither Harris nor Patrick and his colleagues included children in their studies, but Weale and Bradshaw (1980) carried out a special analysis of the General Household Survey to make estimates of the prevalence and characteristics of disabled children. They found a prevalence of 70 chronic physical conditions per 1000 children under 16 and compared this with a rate of 111 per 1000 derived by Pless and Douglas (1971) from the National Survey of Child Health and Development. Weale and Bradshaw also looked at the prevalence of a number of individual conditions; their rates for severe mental handicap and spina bifida compared well with estimates from other studies but they found a very low rate for the prevalence of all severities of

cerebral palsy and suggested that the absence of any medical assessment in the GHS contributes to this.

There have been a number of surveys of the disability and handicap
experienced by patients suffering from specific conditions. These
studies have been based on people known to the services or identified
by general practitioners as having the condition. Johnson and Johnson
(1977) in their study of social services support for multiple sclerosis
patients in the west of Scotland selected their patients from lists
provided by the Multiple Sclerosis Society in Glasgow and the
Institute of Neurological Sciences in Glasgow; Hopkins and Scambler
(1977) interviewed 87% of the adult patients with epilepsy identified
by 17 general practitioners in London. But as Patrick and his colleagues and Bowling and Cartwright (1982) have shown, general
practitioners and those in other services may not be aware of their
patients' disabilities and needs. Another study which illustrates this is
considered next.

The needs of the dying

I have included the needs of the dying in this review mainly because I
think they have been inadequately studied. Yet we all die and in the
period before death needs for care are often great. A study which
looked at this (Cartwright, Hockey and Anderson 1973) showed that
most care took place at home but it was estimated that between a
quarter and three-tenths of hospital bed-days are taken up by people
who will be dead within twelve months (page 79). This survey took as
its starting point a random sample of death certificates relating to
adults aged 15 or over and tried to interview the person who knew
most about the last year of the person's life. Interviews were obtained
for 82%. Since the main reason for failure was a refusal, those whose
deaths were particularly upsetting for relatives may be under-
represented. There was also some evidence that those who had no
close relatives were less likely to be included. In addition, information
about their experiences and views was sought from the general
practitioners of the people who died and questionnaires were completed by 79% of the doctors involved, while 95% of the district nurses
in the twelve study areas were interviewed.

A serious limitation of this study design is that the views and
experiences of the person who died could not be obtained directly. It
gives a picture of what it was like for the relatives and friends to care

for and observe the person in the year before the death. But there is only second hand information about the feelings of the person who died about dying at home or in hospital, and about their knowledge or lack of knowledge about their illness and the prognosis. Nevertheless, in spite of these limitations, the study revealed unmet needs for a variety of services.

Some of these needs were normative – for example the general practitioners thought that more of the elderly people needed long-term nursing care and many of the district nurses felt they could not give their patients all the nursing care that was appropriate or spend time talking to them.

Other needs were felt by the relatives or carers: while 10% of the people who died had had some help from a home help, relatives thought nearly half of these could have done with more such help and a further 14% needed some help of that sort. Bathing services and night care were said to be needed more often, as were services for helping with the care of incontinent people at home.

Two-fifths of those suffering from depression, over half of those with loss of bladder control and a quarter of those with loss of bowel control had not sought any professional advice about the problems. These might be regarded as unmet comparative and also normative needs. The fact that they were not expressed is of relevance to the consideration of the way the services function.

Another need considered in that study was for information. A quarter of the relatives said they had been unable to find out all they wanted to know about the patient's illness and its likely outcome. Most, 86%, of the relatives who had been aware that the person was likely to die were glad that they had known, while just under half, 48%, of those who had not known felt this was best. Considering the people who died, just over a third of them were thought by the people interviewed to have known they were dying, but few, 6%, were thought to have discussed it with anyone. Most relatives felt that the knowledge about the outcome was reasonably given to or withheld from the person who died, but of course it is over this that the views of the person who died were most uncertain.

A number of studies have tackled this problem which presents ethical and emotional as well as methodological problems. Hinton (1980) talked to 80 married people with fatal neoplastic disease. Two-thirds said they recognised they might or would die soon. Just over half, 54%, had spoken to their spouse about this; still fewer, just over a quarter, 28%, to the staff who were caring for them. He concludes that 'many patients with cancer would like greater opportunity to discuss their situation more fully but not always with their doctor'. But the patients in Hinton's study 'were selected as being able and willing to converse easily', a restriction which makes it impossible to generalise from the results, particularly as no indication is given of the proportion rejected on this criterion. Hinton, a professor of psychiatry, did all the interviewing himself, and it is uncertain whether similar proportions of patients would want to talk to other sorts of people.

A different approach was adopted by Jones (1981), a consultant chest physician. In a study of 200 consecutive patients with inoperable bronchial carcinoma 'each was told that, after investigation intended to exclude various named diseases including cancer, they would be given truthful clearance or a firm diagnosis if they cared to ask'. They were also told that if they did not care for medical details there would be no need to ask. Seventeen were excluded for various reasons. Of the others, 90 patients asked for the diagnosis, 93 did not, 'despite being given more than one obvious opportunity'. The 90 who had had their questions answered were 'asked if they regretted having asked'; one did so, ten 'subsequently "denied" what they had been told'. Jones concludes that 'some of the "denials" could be due to an admitted tendency to encourage the hesitant to ask'. One gap in his study is the feelings and beliefs of those who did not ask. What assumptions, if any, did they make about the diagnosis? Were their anxieties increased, lessened or unchanged by being given an opportunity to ask questions which they then rejected? It is a pity that Jones did not attempt to predict those who would ask and those who would not. If it were shown that doctors could not predict this better than by chance then it could be argued that randomised trials were ethical.

These questions and studies illustrate some of the limits of surveys in this field. Studies of the views of dying patients themselves have inevitably been confined to special groups suffering from recognised terminal illness (see also Exton-Smith 1961 and Wilkes 1965). In addition it is not possible to find out how people would have reacted if they had been told something, or to be certain how they would react if they had not been given information they already have, while ethical considerations preclude a randomised control trial on the giving of information about such sensitive areas since professionals generally feel they can do better than chance at identifying those who want and those who do not want this type of information. Once again it may not be feasible to design and carry out the ideal study but helpful insights into patients' needs and preferences for particular types of information can still be obtained from surveys. The study by Cartwright, Hockey and Anderson suggested that few patients who were dying had an opportunity to talk about their illness or prognosis to either relatives or professionals. Hinton's survey indicated that more might appreciate an opportunity to do so. Jones has shown that under particular circumstances about half will avail themselves of an opportunity to ask questions although some of these will reject the information they are given. Critics of surveys might argue that there are other, more appropriate ways of finding out what people want to know. Shands and his colleagues (1951) advise not telling patients more than they ask while Saunders (1969) argues that in caring for the dying 'the real question is not, "What do you tell your patients?", but rather, "What do you let your patients tell you?".' But we need some studies to ascertain the reactions of patients, particularly in a field such as this where the views and practices of the professionals differ quite markedly.

When other sorts of needs are considered – for pain relief, comfort, support, help with personal care and household activities – the experiences of those who have recently died, even though they have to be obtained at second hand, give a picture of the way society cares for people with a wide variety of needs. There is a comprehensive sampling frame, death certificates, which identifies all the dead: studies based on such a sample can claim universality and will reveal unmet needs as well as those which were met.

Urinary incontinence

People suffering from incontinence of urine may need medical help to relieve their condition and/or practical help to cope with the problem. It is generally thought to be an under reported condition (*Lancet* 1977) and surveys have been carried out to determine its prevalence.

One study (Thomas et al 1980) was concerned with 'recognised' and 'unrecognised' incontinence. The survey of 'recognised' incontinence was carried out in two London boroughs by contacting 'relevant agencies' and asking them to provide details of the patients in their care who fulfilled the study definition of urinary incontinence. The sources included community nurses, various institutions, schools, certain voluntary societies and pad and laundry services but not, apparently, general practitioners. This part of the study was confined to people aged 15 and over. Estimated prevalence rates were 0.2% in women aged 15–64 and 0.1% in men of that age range; 2.5% in women and 1.3% in men aged 65 and over.

The survey of 'unrecognised incontinence' covered people aged five and over and was based on the lists of 12 general practitioners in London, Bristol and South Wales. The general practitioners sent postal questionnaires to patients aged 16 and over and 'parents were asked to fill in forms for children aged 5–15'. (In practice mothers were normally sent forms about the children, and fathers only if mothers were not identified. A few children, for whom neither parent could be identified, were omitted.) After two reminders, 89% returned a completed questionnaire.

The report states that for both parts of the study regular urinary incontinence was defined as 'involuntary excretion or leakage of urine in inappropriate places or at inappropriate times twice or more a month, regardless of the quantity of urine lost'. In practice the postal questionnaire to patients refers to circumstances in which people 'wet' themselves.

From the postal inquiry, just over 2% were classed as uncertain, while 3.3% of males and 8.5% of females reported regular incontinence. Age and sex data were presumably available from the practice records. The only other question asked on the postal study – apart from the questions on incontinence – related to the number of babies women had had. This was referred to as parity in the paper.

To validate the questionnaire, 237 patients from two of the study areas or practices who had reported regular incontinence were asked by their general practitioners to agree to be interviewed by one of the survey team nurses. Seventy-five per cent were interviewed and of these 89% were classified as incontinent at the interview. Half of the discrepancies arose through 'temporary causes of incontinence'. It was only the people interviewed who were asked about any help they were receiving from the district nurse, health visitor, social worker, pad service or laundry service. Of the 158 still incontinent when interviewed, only 10% were in touch with these services. But the authors point out it does not necessarily follow that all these patients needed or would have been helped by such services. They also point out that the estimates of prevalence of incontinence obtained from the postal survey and interview follow-up were greater than those obtained from the study of recognised incontinence. And one group not covered by their definition on the postal survey was those patients who would have been incontinent were they not being well managed. They comment that the difference might be due to the under-reporting of recognised incontinence or 'might reflect the selected nature of the practices participating in the . . . survey, where the level of services received by incontinent patients may be greater than in other practices'. It is indeed hard to understand why the two parts of the study were done in different areas when it would have been more illuminating to do them in the same areas. If they had been done in the same areas this might also have provided some clues about possible false negatives on the postal study. No attempt was made to identify these.

Another study by Yarnell et al (1981) was concerned with the prevalence and severity of urinary incontinence among women on the electoral register for 'a defined geographical area in South Wales'. This study was based on interviews – the response rate being 95%. Incontinence was divided into 'urge', 'stress' and 'complex', and classified by the amount of urine lost and the frequency of occurrence. The women were asked about any interference with 'social or domestic' life, and what medical action they had taken. Only 9% of those with incontinence had consulted a general practitioner. They concluded that the prevalence of 'significant' urinary incontinence in the general population of women is between 3.5% and 7.1%, although '45% admitted to some degree of (urinary) incontinence'.

In some ways it may seem inappropriate to regard these studies as relating to needs since they did not attempt to identify particular needs. However they were both concerned with finding out the proportion of the incontinent who were in touch with services; and they can hardly be classified as surveys to identify factors associated with disease since the only characteristic considered by both was age, one study also taking into account sex and parity. Yarnell et al end: 'It is difficult to estimate how much help could be given to these women. Only a small proportion of those affected appear to seek medical help, and this may reflect both reluctance to discuss the condition and a low expectation of benefit from treatment. Further work is clearly needed on . . . the evaluation of existing treatments.'

It is surprising to me that neither study tried to find out anything about the reasons why people do not seek help for such problems, and the sort of help received by people who do get in touch with services.

The answers to the two questions may well be related. Cartwright, Hockey and Anderson found that one of the main reasons for people not consulting about particular problems was a realistic assessment of the probable outcome (page 87). And as the *Lancet* (1977) editorial on incontinence put it: 'Unfortunately, for many the arrival at the outpatient clinic often marks a new start, rather than an end to their problems.'

The people who carried out these studies were clearly concerned about the problems of the incontinent; their surveys may have made more people aware of the extent of the problem but they missed an opportunity to illuminate it in other ways.

Trouble with feet

Two surveys of foot problems were more directly concerned with needs and the ways in which needs might be met. Clarke's study (1969) aimed to 'find out the kinds of trouble people have with their feet, and to estimate the unmet need and unmet demand for professional treatment' (page 7). Two complementary methods of approach were used. First, a random sample of people taken from the electoral register of 12 parliamentary constituencies in England and Wales were interviewed in their homes to find out about their perception of their foot problems, their attitudes to them and their expectation about alleviation. Second, to provide professional diagnoses of people's foot conditions and professional assessments of the need for care, a proportion of the same people were examined by trained chiropodists using a standardised foot examination record. The response rate to the interview study was 82%, and a random half of these were asked if they would be willing to have their feet examined by a chiropodist at home. Only 50% of those asked agreed and had the examination. More of those who were examined had reported foot problems at the interview than of those who were not examined: 72% compared with 58%. This bias has been allowed for in Table 3 which compares the proportion reporting foot problems at interview with those found by the chiropodists at examination.

More people were recorded by the chiropodists as having foot problems than reported it at the interview, 83% compared with 62%. Even so, a third of the people reported some pain or disability because of trouble with their feet. But while the prevalence of foot trouble was high, the proportion receiving professional treatment was low: 14% of

Table 3 Proportion of people with foot troubles reported at interview and found at examination – after correction for bias

	%
No foot trouble at examination or interview	10
Foot trouble at examination but not at interview	28
No foot trouble at examination but some at interview	7
Foot trouble at both examination and interview	55
Number of people (= 100%)	285

those interviewed had had some professional treatment for their feet in the six months before the interview, 9% from a chiropodist. This compares with an estimated 37% assessed by the examiners as needing treatment from a chiropodist – and a further 20% for whom they thought it would be helpful but not essential. The unmet need for care, a normative measure assessed by the chiropodists, exceeded not only the people's demands but their felt needs. This raises some doubt about the relevance of the chiropodists' assessment of need. But the consistency of their assessments had been tested in a small study in which ten elderly people had their feet examined and assessed independently by four different chiropodists – the two who did the survey examinations and two, more experienced, teachers of chiropody. Over their assessment of need for treatment there was complete agreement between the four chiropodists for eight of the ten.

The main reason for the gap between the chiropodists' assessments of need for treatment and the individuals' perceptions of their need was not that people ignored their foot trouble but that they dealt with it by self treatment. One suggestion arising from the study was for a controlled evaluative study of chiropody and self treatment to assess how far people are doing things which are harmful or ineffective and the extent to which chiropodists cure and relieve conditions.

Another survey of foot problems of the elderly was carried out by Ebrahim, Sainsbury and Watson (1981) in four hospital wards 'to establish the prevalence and nature of foot problems among patients in our acute geriatric assessment and rehabilitation wards'. A hundred patients completed a questionnaire about their ability to walk, previous use of chiropody services, ability to cut their own toe nails and whether their feet were painful. 'Patients' answers were confirmed by nursing staff or relatives.' Their feet were examined and footwear inspected. Only one patient had no problems with her feet. The authors conclude: 'The patients surveyed had a high prevalence of foot problems and most were unable to attend to their own foot care. . . . Careful assessment of foot problems is an important part of the examination of the elderly patient. Problems such as nail cutting, dirt and masceration could be dealt with easily without skilled training, but many problems require a chiropodist's attention.'

Methodological issues

The main problems in these surveys have been the identification of appropriate samples, definition of the needs, and validation of the results. There have also been some ethical issues over the formulation of questions.

Sampling Several of the studies have demonstrated the usefulness of a postal screen for identifying groups of people with different types of need. Such an approach makes it possible to include people with unmet needs and not just to confine the survey to people already in touch with services. False positives may be identified at subsequent interviews, but the problem of false negatives is more difficult to deal with. When needs are common, such as those related to foot problems, it is feasible to interview a random sample such as those taken from the electoral register. But for the rarer conditions investigators inevitably have to carry out a postal screen or to depend on professional carers or specific voluntary organisations to identify the sufferers. In the latter instance they may exclude those with unmet needs who are not known to the services or who are not in touch with other organisations. A way of identifying a group of people with a wide variety of needs who may not have been in contact with services is to use death certificates as a sampling frame. It is also possible to draw a sample of people recorded on the death certificate as dying of specific conditions and then study their needs retrospectively, in the same sort of way as Cartwright, Hockey and Anderson (1973) studied a sample of all adult deaths. But using death certificates has the disadvantage of not being able to obtain information from the person who died.

Definition of needs presented difficulties for most of the studies. But the use of an activities of daily living scale, based on ability to perform essential activities unaided, so that severity of disability is proportional to the degree of dependence (Garrad and Bennett 1971) could facilitate comparison between various studies of disability, although most researchers tend to modify existing measures to meet their own requirements.

With specific needs, such as those for foot care or for incontinence services, identification and definition still present problems. Incontinence might be regarded as a specific clinical problem, but the data are clearly far from hard: the level of incontinence reported depends on the precise questions asked and validation is as necessary in this field as in others.

Validation has been attempted in one form or another in several of these studies. Warren (1975) has confronted the issue of differential identification of problems by patients and professional agencies; Jefferys et al (1969) compared responses to questions with performance of physical tests; Warren (1976) checked impaired people's statements about the nature of the underlying medical condition against general practitioners' assessments; Thomas et al (1980) arranged for a group of patients who had reported regular incontinence to be interviewed by a nurse; and Patrick and his colleagues (Peach et al 1980) looked at results from postal and interview-administered questionnaires. Clarke (1969) compared assessments by people about their own foot troubles with those of chiropodists and also considered the consistency of professional assessments. Cartwright, Hockey and Anderson (1973) compared data from interviews and death certificates in relation to cause of death, age at death, place of death and social class. However these validation exercises do not encompass all the problems of sampling and definition. For instance, Warren (1975) in his comparison of a household survey and agency records points out: 'No data are available about those who refused or returned a negative reply [to the household survey] but were not in contact with any service approached. This group could contain severely impaired people who were strongly determined or unwilling to seek any form of statutory or voluntary help.' The validation exercises of Thomas and colleagues identified wrong positives but did not attempt to look for wrong negatives while Cartwright, Hockey and Anderson (1973) only considered the validity of the few characteristics recorded on the death certificate.

In conclusion

The various studies discussed in this chapter have all been concerned with establishing the extent of needs. For the handicapped or disabled the first aim of the studies was to find out the extent of the problem, while some of the Local Authority Surveys took this a step further by trying to identify the needs of individuals. In these instances the surveys were used not so much for research but as a part of actual services. There is a somewhat similar division between the two studies of foot problems. Clarke's survey (1969) was a national one on a random sample of the adult population, aimed at establishing extent of needs in the population, while Ebrahim and his colleagues were concerned with a particular group of patients under their care; when problems were identified they were presumably treated and the results of their study were probably intended to be incorporated directly into management policy. But studies of the incontinent fell between these stools(!): their estimates of the prevalence of incontinence related to particular areas but they did not apparently exploit this by identifying needs in a way which had direct service implications.

The surveys of the dying also demonstrate the two approaches. That of Cartwright, Hockey and Anderson covered a national sample and a variety of needs, trying to show the successes and failures of existing services in meeting these needs. The other two studies of the dying discussed here related solely to needs for information and were carried out by clinicians actively involved in the care of patients to illuminate and guide their own practice and that of their colleagues.

The more 'epidemiological' approach, covering national samples, and the individual area or practice one, are complementary. The random survey puts the problem into perspective and makes it possible to assess the wider implications of the smaller, service based, studies; while the smaller, service orientated surveys, can explore ways of meeting the needs revealed.

5 Use of services

Surveys which address three questions are reviewed in this chapter. The three questions are first: 'Are services reaching those in need?'; second: 'Why do some people in need not use the services?'; and third: 'Who uses services and why?' Finally, an experimental study designed to affect use of services for certain symptoms is described.

Are services reaching those in need?

One way to approach this question is to survey those who have not been in contact with a service to see whether they need it or not. However it is only practicable to use this approach for services needed or used by a high proportion of people and when records are available to identify both the users and non-users in a population. So this approach is seldom used. One exception was a study by Kessel and Shepherd (1965) of people in one practice who had **not consulted their general practitioner** for two years and another group who had not done so for ten years or more. They also contacted a group of recent attenders for comparison. Subjects were interviewed at home and were also asked to complete a health questionnaire, the Cornell Medical Index. Response rates varied from 77% of those who had not consulted their doctor for ten years, to 86% of those who had not done so for just two years and to 90% of the recent attenders. This was after removing 'dead' cards from the practitioner's records.

Both groups of non-attenders contained less young and more old people than the general population. Non-attenders did not take a more limited view of the doctor's role but they were rather more critical of his or her services. They were not neglectful of their health but took a more favourable view of it and worried less about it. Kessel and Shepherd conclude: '. . . broadly speaking those who seldom or never consult their practitioners appeared to be healthy'. They point out that it was done in a single practice in a homogeneous middle-class area. But although it has important implications the only other study I have located of this type (Baker 1976) was also carried out in a single practice, and makes no reference to, or comparisons with, the earlier, Kessel and Shepherd study.

Another study comparing users and non-users was carried out by

Anderson and his colleagues (1977); but they were concerned with the implications for self-care. They matched 60 patients who visited their general practitioner with 60 registered with the same doctor who were of the same sex and in the same ten-year age group and who had not visited the doctor for at least one year, but had recently experienced symptoms similar to those presented by those attending a doctor. To do this matching they had to interview 685 patients, so 82% of the interviews were not used for the comparisons. Because of the matching it is not possible to tell how far use and non-use were related to age, or sex or reported complaints. They found that infrequent users of doctors perceived themselves as healthier than did frequent users. This is consistent with the findings of Kessel and Shepherd, but whereas Kessel and Shepherd found a considerable amount of self-medication among both non-attenders and recent attenders whose habits did not differ in this respect, Anderson and his colleagues reported more self-treatment among the non-users in their study. Such a difference could result from the different approaches adopted.

Another way to approach this problem is to identify people with needs and to find out if they are being cared for appropriately. The question then is similar to the one on need for particular services which was discussed in the previous chapter. Since the object of the exercise is to identify people needing care who are not in touch with services, a sampling frame is needed which does not depend on use of services. So this approach too is only practical for relatively common needs, or for needs that can be identified by a postal screen. Services that have been studied in this way are chiropody and dentistry. Clarke's study *Trouble with feet* (1969), has already been described. The studies of **dentistry** (Bulman et al 1968 and Gray et al 1970) follow a similar pattern so are only discussed briefly. The survey of Bulman and his colleagues was done in two contrasting urban areas. Although the authors refrained from making national estimates from this, others were not so restrained and an estimate of 17 million people in England and Wales with no natural teeth received considerable publicity. The national study by Gray and his colleagues produced a considerably smaller estimate of 13 million. Both studies were based on interview surveys with people drawn at random from the electoral registers followed by a dental examination. In the national study 85% of the selected sample were successfully interviewed and 77% examined, so 91% of those interviewed were also examined. An interesting innovation on this study was a small postal inquiry, two months after the completion of the fieldwork, to find out if participation in the survey had made any impact on dental attendance. This was thought likely as each informant had been given a leaflet recommending that people who had not been to the dentist for a year or more should make an appointment as soon as possible. The authors described themselves as 'fairly surprised that as many as 90% of the people to whom the leaflet referred, had not made an appointment to see a dentist'.

A study which falls roughly in this field, and was concerned with the **broad field of ill-health** was carried out in Bermondsey and Southwark by Wadsworth, Butterfield and Blaney (1971). The stated aim of this survey (page 7) was 'to ascertain the extent of disease . . . in a study population, and to describe the measures taken to alleviate or cure these complaints so that the proportion referred to medical care might be estimated'. A random sample of 2,500 people was selected from the register of electors; the response rate was 87%. The interview began with general, open-ended questions about health; these were followed by check lists of medicines, measures and treatments used in the previous 14 days and then by a check list of complaints experienced in the same period. After that there were two questions on accidents and the late effects of injuries and then one check list of chronic complaints ever experienced and one of disabilities. Information was classified into three groups: symptoms or complaints; diagnoses or causes; medicines and measures. The main finding of the study was 'the great extent of lay diagnosis and treatment, as compared with recourse to medical care' (page 91). The authors did not draw any definite conclusions about needs for care although they compared their results with those from a screening clinic in Southwark. In the study by Wadsworth and his colleagues, 4.9% of people reported no complaints or diseases, while in the Southwark screening study it was 6.7%; and '52% of the persons screened were found to be in need of further investigation and possibly treatment' (page 85). However the Southwark screening study did not involve interviews or questionnaires and so does not meet the criterion of a survey laid down for this review.

Yet another way to find out about people in need but not receiving help from services is to study people who do eventually come into contact with the services – but later than is appropriate from a normative definition of needs. People who do not attend for antenatal care until late in their pregnancy have been studied by McKinlay (1970) and O'Brien and Smith (1981). The speed of diagnosis, referral and treatment in cancer of the breast and large bowel have been studied by MacArthur (1981). She obtained information from general practitioners, from cancer registry forms (containing data abstracted from hospital case notes) but primarily from interviewing each patient in hospital after the disease had been definitively diagnosed and usually treated. She found that the duration of symptoms recorded on the forms for breast cancer patients was shorter than from the patient's description at interview, and concluded that the most likely reason for the discrepancy was that patients had given shorter durations to the doctor taking the case history because they did not want to admit to considerable delay. 'There were fewer symptoms recorded on the form than had been described by the patients in the interview, in particular, inverted nipple and breast discomfort/pain were more often omitted whereas lump was always recorded. It is suggested that either patients describe only the main symptom to the doctor, or the doctor taking the history decides that lump is the main symptom and does not record the other symptoms. If this is the case a false picture of the symptomatology of breast cancer emerges.' In large bowel cancer delay from first medical consultation to referral for specialist opinion was much more significant than in breast cancer. And the factor most closely associated with the speed of referral for specialist opinion was whether the general practitioner examined them at their first visit or not.

Why do some people in need not use services?

This question tends to be asked about preventive and screening services such as antenatal care (Douglas 1948, Illsley 1956, Macintyre 1981), screening for pulmonary tuberculosis (Cochrane 1954, Cartwright, Martin and Thomson 1959), cervical cancer (Sansom et al 1975, Wakefield and Baric 1965) and hypertension (O'Brien and Hodes 1979). I have chosen to discuss a study which asked this question about family planning services, and one which is more unusual in that it relates to a group of people with a variety of problems – the disabled.

In Bone's first study of **family planning services** (1973) she set out 'to describe and assess the adequacy of the existing family planning services in England and Wales and to suggest fruitful lines of development to ensure that everyone needing advice on contraception could obtain it without difficulty'. She sampled 'married women' (including the widowed, divorced, separated and those who said they were cohabiting) aged 16–40 and single women aged 16–35. Response rates were 86% for the married, 77% for the single. To some extent this study broke new ground by including single women in a national study of contraception sponsored by a government department. But although single women were included they were not asked whether they were sexually experienced, because of 'the limitations peculiar to an official inquiry'. Estimating the proportion of single people in potential need of such services and identifying their characteristics would seem to be an essential part of the study's aims. Bone attempted the first. She estimated that between 33% and 38% of unmarried women in that age group were experienced. She did this on the basis of her own data on the proportion (23%) who 'provided evidence of experience' (in almost all cases the evidence was use of contraception), and data from Schofield's (1965) and McCance and Hall's (1972) surveys on the proportion of sexually experienced people in their studies who had used contraception. Schofield's study was carried out in 1964 and covered those aged 15–19; that of McCance and Hall was done later but related solely to unmarried undergraduates at Aberdeen University. Both would appear flimsy ground from which to make such an estimate for single women aged 16–35 in 1972. In Bone's later study, too, (carried out in 1975, published 1978) the single women were not asked about their sexual experience: '. . . it was again felt that the time was not ripe to question single women, and particularly the younger ones, directly about their sexual experience' (page 4). On this study Bone did not attempt to estimate the proportion who were sexually active. But a year after Bone's second study, such questions were introduced for single women in another study carried out in the same organisation (Dunnell 1979), while Farrell (1978) had included similar questions in her national study of 16 to 19 year olds in 1974–5. It is not possible to work out from the published data from Dunnell's study how accurate Bone's estimate was, but by 1976 half the single women aged 16–49 said they were sexually experienced, which suggests that it was possibly an under-estimate.

Bone's study highlighted the various perceived disadvantages of each contraceptive method and some of the problems related to the accessibility and acceptability of clinics and general practitioner services. It did not include men, so the importance of their preferences in determining use and choice of methods and services was not determined directly.

Cartwright's study of parents and family planning services (1970) included mothers, fathers, general practitioners, health visitors and doctors working in family planning clinics. It was based on a sample of legitimate births, so the views of the unmarried were not represented. But by spanning the views of both potential clients of a service and of the professionals providing the service, it highlighted one of the big gaps in services at that time: many mothers because of diffidence or embarrassment wanted to be offered contraceptive advice by their general practitioners while most general practitioners waited to be asked for such advice.

A very different sort of survey which threw light on the question of why people may not use services, was Blaxter's study of the **meaning of disability** (1976). She was concerned to explore the processes of categorisation of disablement and to demonstrate, from the disabled person's point of view, the nature of his or her problems. 'Since processes of definition are a central focus of the study, it was obviously not appropriate to study any group of people already defined as disabled. The sample, therefore, consisted of all those people discharged during a four-month period from four wards of a large teaching hospital, whose illness or accident was neither trivial nor expected to be soon fatal.'* She points out that the categories of 'trivial' and 'poor prognosis' could not be clear-cut. The study was restricted to people of working ages; 16–65. Four of the 205 identified were excluded at the request of their general practitioner and one could not be traced; 97% of the others were interviewed soon after their discharge from hospital and at two to three-monthly intervals throughout the following year.

Blaxter's study suggested that one of the reasons why services for the disabled may be underused is the dilemma for the professionals 'of singling out an undesirable characteristic – physical impairment – without appearing to stigmatize; the dilemma of persuading people to accept a label, "disabled" or "handicapped", which although it may be offered with the intention of helping may be rejected because potential clients find it meaningless, or alternatively because they find it too full of unwelcome meanings' (page 238).

Another explanation for not using specific services may be the lack of a clear clinical label. Blaxter describes (pages 235–6) a young man who had not been told that he was suffering from multiple sclerosis.

---

* This quotation is taken from an unnumbered page in the introduction.

He applied for certain welfare benefits on the grounds of poverty, not ill-health, and did not seek help and support from the self-help Multiple Sclerosis Society. Blaxter maintains that 'his inability to define a legitimate role for himself . . . crucially affected his help-seeking behaviour'.

Who uses services and why?

This question tends to be asked when people are concerned with the maldistribution of care, and particularly with the uneven or inequitable use of care by people in different social classes or geographical areas. These types of studies are discussed elsewhere. Another situation which prompts this question is the suspicion that services may be misused or over used. Accident and emergency services and repeat abortions are two of the services about which this question has been posed.

Accident and emergency services A study by Morgan, Walker, Holohan and Russell (1974) in Newcastle was stimulated by the increasing number of patients attending accident and emergency departments which was said to be placing a severe strain on these services. For their sampling frame they used the current register of new patients in the three hospitals with accident and emergency departments in their study area and took a random sample of one in every 100 patients over a period of three months. Patients who were admitted to hospital and those who had had a road traffic accident were excluded. Of the 254 selected, 91% were interviewed in their homes within 14 days of their first attendance at the hospital. Medical data were extracted from the hospital records by medical practitioners. Information was collected about the route by which patients reached the accident and emergency department, reasons for going to hospital rather than to a general practitioner, and about attitudes and expectations of hospital and general practitioner care. It was found that most patients attended the hospital for the treatment of traumatic injury and did so without consulting their own general practitioner. In their conclusion the authors claim: '. . . our investigation suggests that the present organisation of general practice is an important contributory factor in the decision of many patients to attend hospital as casuals'. This is based on comparisons of the proportion of patients in their study whose general practitioners operated an appointment system with the proportion found on a national inquiry by Irvine and

Jefferys (1971) – 80% against 66% – and the smaller proportion in their study who were in favour of an appointment system when compared with another national study (Bevan and Draper 1967). No adjustments were made for age, sex or social class in these comparisons, nor for the different years in which the studies were carried out. The Irvine and Jefferys study related to 1969, the Bevan and Draper to a period before 1967, while the one by Morgan and his colleagues must have been done sometime between 1971 and 1973 – the actual year is not specified in the article. During this period, appointment systems were becoming much more common. In 1964, 15% of patients had general practitioners with appointment systems; by 1977 this proportion had risen to 75% (Cartwright and Anderson 1981, page 29). Morgan and his colleagues point out that they had investigated only those patients who sought and received treatment from the hospital and they subsequently surveyed patients who had received care for accidental injury from their general practitioners. In a paper reporting on the two phases of the study Russell (1977) reached a different conclusion. Commenting on the view taken by the Expenditure Committee of the House of Commons that the use of appointments systems and deputising services can be thought to have had some influence on patients' decisions to attend AEDs he concluded: 'Not only are these two variables not even remotely associated with the choice of care system, as shown by a simple cross-tabulation, but neither was able to make any contribution to our multivariate statistical analysis.'

As a third part of the study (Holohan, Newell and Walker 1975) 'postal questionnaires were sent to the 285 general practitioners whose patients were known to have attended the accident and emergency department of the three hospitals involved in the earlier study'. The response rate after one reminder was 70%. The results of this part of the study were summed up in another paper (Holohan 1976) as revealing 'no unwillingness to provide treatment for minor injury in general practice'. This conclusion appears to be based on the proportion of the doctors who expressed a willingness to strap sprains, 85%, excise simple cysts, 24%, and stitch cuts, 62%. These proportions were compared with patients' expectations and it was found that patients underestimated the willingness of their doctors to strap sprains and stitch cuts, while over the excision of simple cysts patients' expectations coincided more closely with the reluctance of their general practitioners to undertake treatment.

A number of the conclusions drawn from this series of studies are open to criticism. These stem from an inappropriate study design. If the researchers were concerned with the relationship between general practitioners' appointment systems and patients' use of acident and emergency departments they should have designed their study differently, finding out about the current use of appointment systems in their locality and not relying on comparisons with a national study at a different point in time.

If they wanted to make statements about the willingness or unwillingness of general practitioners to provide treatment for minor injury in their practice, they needed to do more than question general practitioners about whether they usually do three specific procedures – and then apparently ignore the fact that only a quarter of the doctors said they carried out one of these procedures. At the same time they did not analyse further the third of patients who had contacted their general practitioner or the practice receptionist before going to the hospital except to say they delayed longer and more of them were 'non-trauma cases'.

If they posed the question whether the patients' preference for hospital care was a reflection of underlying attitudes in favour of hospital (as they did in the article by Morgan et al), it did not answer it to make a comparison with a national study (Cartwright 1967), show that their patients were more hospital oriented and then state: 'we gained the impression during our interviews that this orientation was related to their recent hospital experience'.

Finally, if they state that the aim of the survey was 'to examine the social and medical characteristics of patients attending accident and emergency departments in three hospitals' (Morgan et al), why did they exclude patients admitted to hospital and those who had suffered a road accident, without either discussing their reasons or giving any figures about the numbers involved?

In my view this study demonstrates a mis-match of objectives and design.

Repeat abortions A number of studies have been done in the United States where multiple abortion is not regarded as an appropriate method of birth control. Rather surprisingly it has received little attention in this country but one study (Brewer 1977) looked at women who had had three or more legal abortions. Brewer argued that 'a study of third-timers might shed more light on the factors involved'.

The study was confined to those having their third or later abortion at a British Pregnancy Advisory Clinic or at either of two private clinics in Birmingham. As the statistics do not distinguish between people having a second and a third (or later) abortion, there were some problems in identifying all those who were eligible for inclusion in the study and 'some women left the clinics before an interview could be arranged'. There is no information about the number missed nor about the proportion who were unwilling to participate. 'All patients were interviewed after their abortion on the day of operation, to minimize the likelihood that they might conceal or embellish certain information in the belief that their chances of getting an abortion might be adversely affected.' Information was obtained about the women's age, marital status, number of 'full-term pregnancies', education, use of contraception and 'any past history of medical consultations for emotional disorder'.

Among the first 50 patients seen, 23 had experienced a contraceptive method failure while 24 had been erratic in their use of contraception. These two categories were carefully and stringently defined. For three women their circumstances had changed substantially between conception and abortion. More of those classified as erratic contraceptors than of the contraceptive failures had had a previous consultation for a psychiatric disorder. 'A number of abortions in the method failure group might have been avoided had these women obtained other and better contraceptive methods. Four women had requested sterilisation, but had been refused, and three had unsuccessfully requested a coil, between the latest, and the previous abortion. . . . There were too many women who were advised repeatedly to use the oral contraceptive in spite of their resistance, and perhaps without adequate discussion of alternative methods. Ten of the erratic group were using the oral contraceptive.'

Comparisons are made of the marital status of this group with BPAS patients as a whole. But unfortunately Brewer made no estimate of the proportion of abortion patients having their first, second or third abortion. In spite of this he concluded: '. . . although the incidence of second-time abortion indicates that the human capacity for wishful thinking is considerable, the difficulty experienced in collecting sufficient third-timers for this study suggests that it is not infinite'. Apparently it took him over three years to obtain his 50 patients.

An experimental study designed to affect use

This study was developed from an earlier one in a London group practice (Morrell, Gage and Robinson 1971). This had apparently shown that in children under the age of 16 six symptoms – stuffy or running nose, sore throat, cough, vomiting, diarrhoea and minor trauma – accounted for over half the new requests for medical care. As a result of this finding, 'a simple 16-page booklet illustrated with cartoons describing how these symptoms can be managed at home and when it is appropriate to seek medical care' was prepared and its effect evaluated by a randomised control trial (Anderson, Morrell, Avery and Watkins 1980). The results showed that the study group who received the booklet demanded significantly fewer home visits compared with the controls who did not. They also requested significantly fewer surgery consultations for three of the six symptoms. The survey part of the study was designed to test the hypothesis that 'patients who received the booklet would, when interviewed three months after the end of the study, show better knowledge of the management of the symptoms described in the booklet than the central group.' Interviewing was done by a health visitor who did not know whether the patients were in the study or control group until she had obtained answers to the last few questions. The survey showed that 'the booklet did not lead to any increase in knowledge in the mothers receiving it . . . [but] 76% of the mothers had consulted the booklet at some time in the year of the study and 28% . . . in the three months before the interview'. The authors conclude that the 'fall in the new requests for care for the symptoms described in the booklet . . . may be interpreted as indicating that what patients need to respond appropriately to common symptoms of illness is a simple reference manual rather than an educational programme designed to increase their knowledge about the management of illness'. But they include a warning: 'A more disturbing possibility is that the booklet had a non-specific effect in deterring patients from consulting the doctor.' An analysis of consultation rates for three symptoms *not* described in the booklet showed no significant differences between the study and control groups for two of the three but for the third the study group had significantly fewer consultations initiated by patients. (Morrell, Avery and Watkins 1980).

Methodological issues

A variety of methodological problems were identified in the studies discussed in this chapter:

1 Lack of replication or comparisons for a study of non-attendance based in a single practice (Kessel and Shepherd).
2 The waste of data involved in identifying and matching patients with similar conditions who had and had not consulted their doctors about them (Anderson et al 1977).
3 Drawing conclusions about the under-use of services from data about the gap between lay diagnosis of ill-health and recourse to services (Wadsworth, Butterfield and Blaney).
4 Constraints and inhibitions about asking single women about their sexual experience (Bone).
5 A mismatch between aims and methods in a group of studies about accident and emergency services.
6 Considering only an extreme of a variable and not trends with increasing intensity. (Brewer 1977).

There were two other interesting methodological observations. One study demonstrated the lack of effect of a survey about dentistry on consultation with dentists (Gray et al). Another showed the superiority of interviews with patients over doctors' records in providing information about symptoms and their duration (MacArthur).

In conclusion

Many studies have been done on the use of services. Alderson and Dowie (1979) list 109 in their review, but four of the ten studies discussed in some detail in this chapter were not included in their review, mainly because they were published later. So it is a field which attracts much work and interest because it tends to identify gaps in existing services and to indicate ways in which services might reach more people in need, or help them more appropriately.

A feature of two or three surveys reviewed was that although they focused on people using one type of service they revealed inadequacies in another service. MacArthur's interviews with patients in hospital highlighted some failures in general practice; Brewer's survey of women having three or more abortions pinpointed some of their difficulties in obtaining adequate advice and help about contraception. It may be easier for researchers to gain access to study patients in one service setting if it is felt that the shortcomings they are likely to identify relate to another service. But any recommendations arising from the research may have less chance of being implemented simply because the relevant people are less likely to be aware of them.

6 *Effects and side effects of care*

There are three basic ways in which surveys have been used to study the effects of care: first by comparative studies of different types of care, secondly by comparisons of people who are given a particular form of care with those who receive no care and thirdly by follow-up studies of patients who have been cared for in specific ways. Comparisons of different types of care, and of care versus no care, are sometimes made by clinical trials: patients in two groups may be matched by known characteristics believed to affect the outcome (or sometimes to interact with the treatment), or they may be allocated at random. The trial may be 'blind', in which case the patient is unaware which treatment, or non-treatment, he or she is receiving; ideally it is 'double-blind' when neither the patient nor the doctor administering the treatment knows. Often the outcome indicators are precise and limited. Many clinical trials do not involve surveys but it would often be better if they did, so that other extraneous effects of care could be identified and assessed. Without such surveys the care givers are likely to be unaware of some of the many different ways in which treatment may affect people's lives – the limitations on their work, leisure activities, diet; the physical and psychological symptoms and other changes in their habits, self-image and life styles.

In this chapter I start by describing a controlled trial, which included an interview survey, of two methods of treatment.

A controlled trial: the management of stroke in the elderly

This study compared the management of elderly patients with acute stroke in a specialist stroke unit and in medical units. The study was designed to test the hypothesis that 'the proportion of patients who could be returned to independence after admission to a stroke unit would be higher than that of patients who were admitted to medical units' (Garraway, Akhtar, Smith and Smith 1981). They used what they refer to as the 'concept of triage' ('the action of assorting according to quality' – Shorter OED) to divide patients aged 60 or more with a first stroke into three bands, 'upper', 'middle' and 'lower' – 'using selection criteria derived from previous studies of the natural history of stroke'. Only those in the middle band were included in the study – so those who were likely to do poorly whether they were rehabilitated or not and those likely to recover spontaneously without rehabilitation were excluded from the trial. Once eligibility had been established, patients were allocated at random to the two treatment groups, one being admitted directly to the stroke unit, the other referred immediately to the Emergency Bed Bureau for placement in a medical unit. The fact that the study was confined to patients for whom outcome was thought likely to be affected by treatment not only increased the probable sensitivity of the study, but also meant that relatively few eligible patients were lost, since before the study started it was found that 80% of what would have been eligible patients were referred to hospital through the Emergency Bed Bureau compared with 42% of those with a poor prognosis and 53% of those with a good one. Nevertheless only 71% of those eligible were referred to the study. This estimate is based on case listings of all stroke admissions in Scottish Hospital Inpatient Statistics and an examination of a random one-in-three of these medical records. This procedure revealed that only 18% of those with a poor prognosis were referred to the study and 23% of those with a good prognosis. The eligible, in the middle band, accounted for 24% of strokes among those aged 60 and over.

The outcome of the acute phase of rehabilitation was assessed on discharge or 16 weeks after admission by an 'activities of daily living unit'. Preliminary results (Garraway, Akhtar, Prescott and Hockey 1980) showed that delay before starting treatment was significantly shorter in the stroke unit than in the medical units and that a significantly higher proportion of the patients admitted to the stroke unit were assessed as independent at the end of the acute phase: 50% compared with 32% of those admitted to medical units.

The authors pointed out that the mean amount of treatment, both for physiotherapy and occupational therapy, received by patients in the stroke unit was significantly less than that received by patients in medical units. But they made no attempt to control for length of stay, which was much shorter in the stroke unit (a mean of 55 days) than in the medical ones (mean 75 days). They concluded: 'These preliminary results are sufficiently encouraging to suggest that several stroke units should be commissioned in various parts of the country and attempts made to replicate the results.'

Sensibly they carried out a follow-up, visiting patients at monthly intervals after discharge or 16 weeks after admission. At these follow-ups they administered an 'index of nursing dependency' and found that 'the initial improvement in outcome brought about by the stroke unit, as shown by the increased proportion of patients assessed as independent at discharge, had disappeared by one year, with 56 patients (55%) from the stroke unit being reassessed as independent compared with 52 (57%) of the patients discharged from medical units' (Garraway, Akhtar, Hockey and Prescott 1980). They put forward two factors that might have contributed to this disappointing result. First: 'A larger number of patients assessed as independent at discharge from the stroke unit subsequently regressed to functional dependence compared with patients discharged from medical units.' And they reckon this may have happened because of 'overprotection by the families of patients who had been treated in the stroke unit'. In fact, as Twining and Chapman (1980) pointed out, the proportion of patients who were independent at discharge but dependent at follow up was 19% of the stroke unit patients compared with 11% of those from medical units – a difference that might have occurred by chance. The significant difference arose among those who were dependent at discharge: whereas only 6% of those discharged from stroke unit subsequently became independent this proportion was 24% among the dependent patients discharged from medical units. The second explanation put forward by Garraway and his colleagues is that: 'This group had stayed in hospital for a much shorter period than other patients in the medical units. Consequently they received less physio- therapy and occupational therapy and we postulate that their full rehabilitation potential had not been realised when they were dis- charged from hospital.' The mean duration of hospital stay was 47 days for these patients and Garraway and his colleagues contrast this with a mean length of stay of 91 days for patients from medical units whose outcome did not change. They conclude: 'The results of the follow-up do not negate the potential improvement in the manage- ment of acute stroke in the elderly that might arise from establishing stroke units. They do, however, confirm that management of stroke continues well beyond the acute phase in hospital.'

A further report on the use of hospital and community services during the follow-up (Garraway, Walton, Akhtar and Prescott 1981) showed that 'no overall difference occurred between stroke unit and medical unit patients in hospital bed days used throughout the study'. It also suggested that 'whatever criteria were used to allocate com- munity (but not hospital) services did not take into account the functional performance of patients'. The authors found this last a surprising finding that 'emphasizes the importance of establishing more precise guidelines for the use of community services in the long-term management of stroke'.

Not all parts of the study fall within the definition of a survey for this review but the outcome assessments and the information about contacts with services involved the questioning of patients or relatives, so by my criteria they can be regarded as surveys. Indeed the methods, being somewhat borderline, are of particular interest. While patients were living at home, data about their contacts with any member of the community health or personal social services were obtained by a log book kept by patients or their relatives, the details being checked for completeness at monthly intervals when the nursing dependency index was administered. This last activity was performed by a nurse and involved monitoring progress in the performance of 20 selected activities of daily living and measuring the level of patient dependency in these activities. There was no set questionnaire, the items were scored on the basis of defined categories.

This was a controlled trial, imaginatively and broadly conceived and involving a multi-disciplinary team consisting of an epidemiologist, a medical statistician, a nursing research director and a physician in geriatric medicine. It has a complex design and its strengths and its weaknesses seem to stem from this complexity. My main comments are centred on two aspects of the design: the selection of patients and the stage at which assessments were made.

First, the selection. My criticism is of the way the data were presented from a scientific viewpoint. In the preliminary results of the trial and in the report on the follow-up (Garraway, Akhtar, Prescott and Hockey 1980 and Garraway, Akhtar, Hockey and Prescott 1980) there was no mention of the fact that the trial was confined to the 24% of patients who were most likely to benefit from care. Yet the first report after commenting that 'admission to the stroke unit did not result in the intensive treatment that might have been implied by the creation of such a unit' and making comparisons with the amount of treatment reported by other workers, concludes with the statement that the 'preliminary results are sufficiently encouraging to suggest that several stroke units should be commissioned in various parts of the country'. No information about the selection of patients was published until eleven months later (Garraway, Akhtar, Smith and Smith 1981).

Turning to the stage at which assessments were made, this led to a lack of comparability between the two groups in this respect. 'The outcome of the acute phase of rehabilitation was assessed when discharge was imminent *or** at a cut-off point of 16 weeks after admission' and the follow-up lasted for a period of one year. However the 'mean duration of hospital stay was 55 days in the stroke unit and 75 days in medical units'. It is stated that this difference arose because more patients in the medical units stayed beyond 16 weeks – but apart from that there is no information in the first two papers about the distribution of stay and therefore no data about the points in time at which the two groups were assessed.

Mean durations of stay are unsatisfactory since they are likely to be greatly affected by a few patients who stay in hospital a long time. In a later paper (Garraway, Walton, Akhtar and Prescott 1981) figures are given which make it possible to calculate that 11% of the stroke unit patients were still in the unit 16 weeks after admission compared with 31% of those in the medical units. So the patients admitted to the stroke unit were on average assessed at an earlier stage than those admitted to hospital units. This makes the difference between the two groups in the proportion assessed as independent at the end of the acute phase of rehabilitation more impressive. But it complicates both the interpretation of services received while in hospital, since different lengths of time are involved, and the assessment of the follow-up period, since what is being compared relates to different periods after the stroke. There is no attempt to control for the differences, although the authors clearly realised that they influenced the services patients received in hospital. For example they simply state that: 'Patients in medical units who received physiotherapy had a significantly longer period of treatment [than those in the stroke unit] and significantly more hours of treatment. These last two differences occurred because the mean duration of hospital stay was longer for patients in medical units.' (Garraway, Akhtar, Prescott and Hockey 1980). It is less certain that they recognised the problem in relation to the follow up, although clearly the follow up period started – and finished – earlier on average for the stroke unit patients. Garraway, Walton, Akhtar and Prescott (1981) comment that: 'A greater use of services amongst stroke unit patients occurred at the beginning of the follow up period with the use of almost all services converging as the follow-up proceeded.' In their discussion they suggest that 'better levels of communication with

* My italics.

general practitioner and community services, combined with the higher level of hospital follow-up arranged prior to hospital discharge must have been contributory factors.' It would be interesting to re-analyse their data controlling for the length of time since the stroke occurred, to see if the differences between the two groups still persisted.

Other points relate to the outcome measurements. Neither of the assessments – the activities of daily living and the nursing dependency index–was made blind. It would have been impossible to make blind assessments for the patients still residing in the initial units during the follow up period, but it might have been possible to do this for the assessments made at the activities of daily living unit or at home.

One puzzle is that the two measures produced such different results: the activities of daily living assessment, made as 'the end of the acute phase of rehabilitation' by the research occupational therapist, showed that more of the stroke unit patients were independent. The subsequent measures of nursing dependency found that the initial advantage disappeared. Yet there was a common core of seven basic activities in both these measures. One possibility is that for some reason the patients from the stroke unit performed better in the inevitably artificial conditions of the activities of daily living unit but no better in the more natural circumstances in which nursing dependency was assessed. It would have been useful to have a controlled comparison of the seven basic activities that were common to the two assessments.

This study illustrates the many ethical, organisational and methodological problems of doing a controlled trial of a particular form of care. It was ambitious and praiseworthy to attempt it. I feel it is somewhat marred by a flaw in the design which might have been overcome in the analysis. Another criticism is of the way the results were initially presented which seems to me to have been misleading.

Some further comparative studies

Another study of **specialised care units**, this time comparing home care with coronary care units for patients with acute myocardial infarction was carried out by Mather et al (1971). This randomised control trial was accepted as ethical because of quoted but unpublished observations by Wright that patients developing myocardial infarction were treated in hospital and at home in about equal numbers and that the mortality rates in the two groups were similar. Only 28% of patients were included in the random trial (9% receiving elective home care and 63% elective hospital treatment) but the mortality rates of the random group were similar for home and hospital treatment: 9.8% for the former, 14.2% for the latter. Since mortality was the outcome measure no interview survey was included in the study. Yet patients' preferences should surely be taken into account in making decisions about different forms of care. The lack of any such assessment was additionally unfortunate in this instance since 'the simplest hypothesis to explain the results is that some people become so frightened by removal from home into coronary care units (and/or hospitals) that cardiac arrest is more frequent than when they are at home' (Cochrane 1972, page 52). Although interviews could have been carried out only with a biased group – the survivors – they might nevertheless throw some light on the extent and nature of such fears and this would add weight to Cochrane's interpretation and possibly suggest ways of reducing such fears or minimising their effects. It might be that certain types of patients who were prone to such anxieties could be identified.

A field in which a number of controlled studies have been done which effectively compare care and no care is **tonsillectomy.** Cochrane (1972) cites three trials (McKee, 1963, Mawson, Adlington and Evans 1967 and Roydhouse 1969) which covered children for whom the value of the operation was considered equivocal. Cochrane concludes: 'Taken altogether the evidence superficially is in favour of the operation but unfortunately two major criticisms can be made against all three.' His two criticisms were, first, that comparisons were made between 'operation' and 'no or inadequate medical treatment', whereas the correct comparison would have been between the 'best surgical' and 'best medical' treatments. Secondly, the assessments were made on parents' statements and opinions and of course the parents knew whether or not the child had had the operation or not. Cochrane argues that the continuous popularity of the operation suggests that most parents believe that tonsillectomy is a cure for upper respiratory disease in children and therefore parents in the control group will have tended to exaggerate the frequency and severity of their child's illness in comparison with parents of a child who has had the operation.

Another controlled trial looked at the effect of **general practitioners' advice against smoking** (Russell, Wilson, Taylor and Baker

1979). Cigarette smokers attending the surgeries of 28 general practitioners during a four week period were assigned (according to the day on which they attended, which was rotated) to one of four groups: two controls and two intervention ones. The latter were both advised by their doctor to stop smoking and one group was also given an information leaflet on how to give up smoking and told that they would be followed up. These two intervention groups and one of the controls were asked to complete a questionnaire about their smoking habits and attitudes before they saw the doctor, and another short questionnaire immediately after seeing the doctor. All four groups were followed up by postal questionnaire one month after their attendance and again one year later. Response rates were 88% at the monthly follow up, and 73% at the yearly. The proportion who filled in the initial questionnaires at the surgery is not given.

The proportion who stated they had given up smoking at the time of the one month follow up was 3.0% in both control groups, 4.6% among those who were given advice only and 7.5% among those given advice, a leaflet and a warning about follow-up. At the one year follow-up the proportions said to be not smoking were 10.3% and 14.0% in the two control groups, 16.7% among those given advice only and 19.1% among those given advice, leaflet and warning.

In the discussion the authors concluded that any general practitioner who adopted the simple routine when consulted by adult patients who smoked of giving them a leaflet, advising them to give up smoking, and warning them that they would be followed up, would have 25 long-term successes in a year.

These results have been used extensively in advertisement in the *British Medical Journal* for Nicorette (a nicotine chewing gum) and they have been widely quoted as evidence that 'general practitioners can be very effective in giving advice or help about habits such as smoking' (Taylor 1982, *British Medical Journal* leader). One major reservation about the study is the lack of validation of the stated changes in smoking habits. It is said in the report that for 14 of those who claimed to have given up smoking the nicotine concentration in their saliva was measured and the observed values were consistent with their claim in all but one. But it is admitted that selection of these patients was inadequate. In addition the numbers were obviously too small and there was no attempt to see whether inappropriate claims were more likely to be made by those who had been advised by their doctors to give up smoking. I would have thought it would have been more useful to follow up those who said they had given up smoking by interview in their homes, asking about the problems they had encountered in doing this and thus giving interviewers an opportunity to assess the validity of their claim. Since the follow up letters were sent by the doctor who had advised those in the intervention groups to give up smoking there may well have been some who were reluctant to admit that they had not followed the advice.

Without validation of this sort, or replication of the study with some built in validation, I do not think the results should be accepted uncritically.

Another reservation relates to the way the authors multiplied the effect of action in one week by 50 to estimate the effect in a year. This seems unrealistic since it assumes that a doctor will be initiating advice to give up smoking to as many patients at the end of the year as at the beginning, whereas of course many of the patients seen at later stages will be the same as the ones who consulted earlier. It would be more appropriate to multiply by 50 and divide by 4, since people consult their general practitioner about four times a year on average. They do not say how, in the study itself, they dealt with smokers who consulted more than once in the study period.

Follow up studies

Follow up studies of patients undergoing surgery or receiving particular forms of care do not usually have specific hypotheses. They are not making comparisons but finding out how the patients are faring in the hope that this will provide clues about the appropriateness of the intervention or about ways in which the treatment might be modified or after-care be more helpful and supportive. Because of the lack of comparisons and hypotheses it may not initially appear to be a particularly useful or fruitful approach; I think such an assessment is erroneous and that this type of study can be useful and revealing. One study was undertaken 'to find out the effects of a permanent colostomy in daily life and to define areas of unmet need which could be attributed to the colostomy' (Devlin, Plant and Griffin 1971). The survey covered all patients with anorectal cancer admitted to the care of two surgical firms and comparisons were made between those who had colostomy operations and those with restorative operations. Patients were interviewed twice, once in outpatients where they had a thorough physical examination, and once in their homes. Questions covered housing, employment, diet, sexual activity, method of evacuation and numbers of actions daily, medical appliances, psychological disturbance, social isolation, hospital experience and utilisation of medical care and social services. Some of the problems revealed by the survey were:

1 A third of the homes of colostomy patients lacked at least one of the basic facilities of an indoor lavatory, a bath and hot water. Although substandard housing tends to make colostomy management more difficult, it seemed that in allocating housing on preferential health grounds local authorities took a narrower view of health hazard than is suggested as reasonable in the study.

2 Most colostomy patients were found to be using 'natural evacuation methods of control' but 36% of these appeared to be unable to control their colostomies.

3 The number of people taking medication to control their colostomy activity bore little relation to the need for this.

4 Of the 28 patients with frequent colostomy actions only eight wore a colostomy bag. 'There appeared to be no reason why these people should not be getting better care except for a lack of communication between the patient and the health and social services.' (Devlin, Plant and Griffin 1971).

5 After discharge from hospital half of the men and over a third of the women complained of urinary trouble such as frequency of micturition, urgency or dysuria.

6 Comparisons with another study (Kinsey, Pomeroy and Martin 1948) indicated a high degree of sexual dysfunction after surgery and especially after colostomy operations. (It is an indication of the lack of survey data in this field that comparisons had to be made with such an old study, from another country and one that was not based on a random sample!)

7 What the authors describe as 'a crude indication of psychological disturbance' suggested that nearly a quarter of those with colostomies were depressed. At least two had committed suicide.

8 Fifty-one per cent of the colostomy patients aged 65 or more scored as socially isolated compared with 10% in a sample survey of old people in a London borough (Townsend 1957).

9 Despite the lack of expertise of the colostomy patients in managing their stoma and their unhealed perineal wound, only 36% said they had been examined by their general practitioner since discharge

from hospital. And the district nurse had visited slightly less than half the colostomy patients.

Following this survey the Joint Board of Clinical Nursing Studies introduced courses for stoma care nurses and the DHSS (1978) issued guidelines to health authorities on stoma problems. The study has other implications. Devlin and his colleagues concluded: 'Society has determined that life must be saved at all costs, and the skill of the surgeon is directed towards this end. We have shown that it is now time to look more closely at the costs and at those who bear them. Far more emphasis must now be placed on the quality of the life saved.'

Another follow-up study of people who had been operated on was carried out on a national basis. Lowdon, Stewart and Walker (1966) identified 1,167 patients who had had a splenectomy in 1961 by a direct approach to all senior administrative medical officers and professors of surgery in England and Wales. A postal follow-up was carried out by obtaining information from family doctors and hospital consultants. Details were obtained for 96% of those identified. The study confirmed that pnemococcal septicaemia and other fulminating infections sometimes follow splenectomy and the authors conclude that it should be avoided whenever possible during the first four years of life.

In practice surgeons were becoming increasingly and uncomfortably aware of the quality of life following some of their more 'heroic' innovations. Lorber, in two retrospective studies (1971 and 1972) of unselectively treated children with spina bifida cystica, identified a set of adverse criteria which if present at birth was associated with an unfavourable prognosis. And he concluded that 'massive effort has led to much avoidable suffering at an exorbitant cost in manpower and money' (Lorber 1972). Since then he has adopted a policy of selective treatment of newborn infants with spina bifida cystica. A follow up study (Lorber and Salfied 1981) showed that the quality of life of the survivors was much higher when compared with that of the previous unselected services in the same unit. Twenty-three per cent of the selected series were still rated as having severe handicaps but this compared with 34% and 50% in the unselected series. All the 71 untreated children died. They were given normal nursing care with feeds on demand but they were not tube fed or treated with antibiotics. Twenty-eight per cent survived for one month, 3% for a year.

Another paediatrician, Zachary (1977), does not believe in selection and takes a different view of the quality of life of the unselectively treated survivors: 'Some have been regarded as living completely miserable and unhappy lives. Yet when I see them I find them happy people who can respond to concern for their personal welfare.'

This controversy raises ethical as well as methodological questions. To what extent is it appropriate to leave such judgements to individual clinicians or to the ethical views of the medical profession? It is probably inevitable that some part of the decisions will depend on the moral values of individual doctors, but these decisions should surely be based on surveys which portray the experiences and attitudes of patients and of the families and others who care for them. It would appear that Lorber has done this in relation to experiences but has not tackled the more difficult one of attitudes. And surveying attitudes in this situation raises other ethical problems.

One study which attempted to do this was carried out recently by Shepperdson (in draft). She attempted to identify children with Down's syndrome born in 1964–65 and 1973–75 and still living with their parents. This was done through schools for the educationally subnormal and through educational psychologists to check on children in normal schools. In 1972, when the first group of parents were initially interviewed, Shepperdson says that euthanasia was 'judged to be too sensitive to be discussed with all parents'. She felt that open discussion was possible by 1981 although there was still some concern about broaching the topic. Shepperdson said that she did not press parents unless she was sure they were willing to answer and three of the 77 were not asked about euthanasia. *The Times* became interested in the study and in a report (21 8 81) stated that '22% of the younger sample were prepared to accept Down's babies as candidates for euthanasia compared with 40% of the older sample'. But Shepperdson in her draft report points out that differences between the two samples did not reach the level of statistical significance although she goes on to say that 'there was a clear trend for parents of the younger children to be less ready to consider Down's syndrome children as candidates for euthanasia'. There was however a statistically significant difference by social class: proportionally more parents in Social Classes I and II than in III, IV or V being in favour of euthanasia for Down's syndrome children.

Another follow-up study of a more straightforward but neglected area was carried out by Beer, Goldenberg, Smith and Mason (1974).

They looked at the ambulance service to an outpatient physiotherapy centre, interviewing the patients during a five-day session to obtain details about their ambulance journeys. At the end of the treatment session each patient was given a stamped addressed postcard and asked to record the time at the end of their treatment, the time of departure of the ambulance from the centre and the time of their arrival home. Complete information was obtained for 86% of the attendances. Using the same methods they studied a further five-day period after the results of the first survey had been discussed with the ambulance staff. So this could also be described as an 'action research project'. The mean waiting time at the centre in the morning sessions declined from 55 minutes in the first period studied to 38 minutes in the second, and the travelling time for the afternoon session fell from 70 minutes to 53 minutes, but there were no significant changes in the average waiting times at home (around 50 minutes), in the travelling time for the morning sessions (an average of 54 minutes) or in the waiting times at the afternoon sessions (just over 30 minutes). 'A few attendances (11 out of 190) were made by more disabled ("non-walking") patients.' For them, 'a total journey time, with waiting, of eight hours was by no means exceptional'. The study showed that 'a quarter of the patients were treated three or more times a week and over half were over 65 years of age'. The authors concluded:

'For these elderly patients, often with dependent spouses, frequent out-patient physiotherapy sessions with the concomitant early starts and frustrating waits can be very disturbing. . . . For some conditions the effectiveness of out-patient physiotherapy is not proved. Then doctors ordering it should remember that it may be merely a potentially socially disruptive placebo.'

Another response might have been a demand for an improvement in transport arrangements.

I am uncertain whether the studies showing the effectiveness of out-patient physiotherapy for certain conditions took into account the side-effects of out-patient attendances. Certainly they should do so, as should studies of other treatments which involve frequent attendances and journeys which are difficult for patients in any way.

A follow-up study in general practice was reported recently (Wright 1982). The doctor noticed that he seemed to be seeing more and more women who had been sterilised and that more women were consulting because of menstrual problems. He wondered if the two changes were related and also whether more women in the practice had been sterilised or whether he was seeing an unrepresentative group. To answer these questions he used his age-sex register, which he described as having been 'set up more as an act of faith than with any specific research project in mind', to identify a random sample of 250 women in the child-bearing years. He also identified 387 sterilised women from his practice records and sent them a postal questionnaire. All but 12, 97%, responded, and were invited to attend for interview. There were no refusals and all but seven, who had left the district before they could be seen, attended. Postal questionnaires were sent to the group of non-sterilised women, matched for age but not parity.

Wright found far more sterilised patients than he had expected – 19% of all married women. From the interviews it appeared that 79% were 'very happy about their sterilisation and had no regrets', 12% had mixed feelings but felt that on balance the operation had been worthwhile, 9% were dissatisfied and unhappy. He compared this relatively high proportion of patients with some regrets with that found on other studies and suggested that the proportion expressing regrets rose with the proportion responding to the various studies. He quoted two studies with response rates of 34% and 35% which found regrets among 1% and 4%, three studies with response rates between 74% and 86% and regrets among 14%–15%, and his own 97% response rate and regrets among 21%. This is an interesting hypothesis but needs careful examination – the particular questions posed, the circumstances of the follow ups, and of course the initial acceptance and counselling of patients for sterilisation all need to be considered as possible reasons for the variation. And the findings from other studies also need to be considered. For instance, Cooper, Gath, Rose and Fieldsend (1982) had a 96% response rate at 18 months follow-up and report some dissatisfaction among 11% which does not fit into Wright's hypothesis so well.

Another of Wright's findings was that 45% of the sterilised group reported current menstrual problems compared with 19% of the matched controls. 'When oral contraceptive users are excluded from the matched group the differences remain statistically highly significant and not dependent on parity.' His final comment, addressed to fellow general practitioners is: 'Do remember, above all, that research should be enjoyable and interesting. Try it!'

Some methodological pitfalls

A number of methodological pitfalls have been identified in these studies of the effects and side effects of care. These relate to the study design, the calculation of estimates, the validation of outcome measures and the presentation of results.

The study design A basic issue in comparative studies of care is the selection of appropriate groups for comparison. Cochrane (1972) maintained that this was not done for the studies of tonsillectomy and that the comparisons should have been between two sorts of care rather than between one form of treatment and no treatment. This surely depends on the somewhat nebulous concept of 'standard practice'. What are the usual alternatives to the treatment under study? If the choice is between two types of treatment has one already been clearly demonstrated to be an improvement on no treatment? If not, it may be necessary to compare three groups: two treatment and a no treatment one. And if no treatment is to be compared with some treatment it will often be appropriate to give a placebo to those not receiving the active treatment.

The calculation of estimates There were two problems with this. In the controlled trial of the management of stroke the estimates of independence and the comparison of services received for the two groups were made at different average lengths of time after the stroke so were not directly comparable. In the controlled trial of the effect of general practitioners' advice against smoking the numbers seen in one week were multiplied by 50 to estimate the effect in a year, which led to an inflated estimate of the effect.

Validation Neither the stroke study nor the one on general practitioners' advice on smoking validated their outcome measures. Ideally in the study on stroke some assessments of patient dependency should have been carried out independently by more than one assessor and although a nurse and a research occupational therapist were both involved in making assessments they did not apparently assess any of the same patients at the same stage. Certainly no measure of their congruence was reported. Some validation of patients' claims to have given up smoking after being advised to do so by their general practitioners seem essential, particularly as it was the same general practitioners who were asking about changes in their smoking habits. Lack of validation throws doubt on the conclusions drawn from the study.

Presentation Failure to point out that the stroke study was confined to the 24% of patients most likely to benefit from treatment could well have misled people quite seriously about the generality of the findings.

In conclusion

The study of the effects and the side effects of care is a field in which surveys have been under used. Cochrane (1972) has argued persuasively for the wider use of randomised controlled trials to evaluate therapy. 'Recent publications using this technique have given ample warning of how dangerous it is to assume that well-established therapies which have not been tested are always effective.' (page 29). I would argue that surveys of the effects of care on patients need to be done in an open and unbiased way in order to reveal the unexpected effects of care and to identify such side effects as fear, anxiety, unrealistic expectations, discomforts, delays and exhaustion. It is not only the effects of specific treatment that need to be studied in this way but the effect of diagnostic procedures, of screening programmes and of such aspects of care as travel to hospital and the disorientating effects of being admitted to hospital. Surveys could also be used more to contribute to a picture of the quality of life of particular groups of patients and this is needed to help assess the value in both human and economic terms of some of the interventions and lack of intervention currently practised.

Although randomised control trials may be the ideal way of evaluating types of care, there are many ethical and methodological problems in setting them up and evaluating the results. More straightforward follow up studies which describe the unwanted as well as the desired effects of care, can be illuminating and helpful. Without such studies we are inevitably ignorant of the implications of much surgical, medical and nursing care. And we should be aware of inappropriate and over-simplified measures of benefit or outcome. Treatment as well as disease often has many effects. It may be tempting to consider single, clearly-defined, measures of outcome, but surveys can reveal other side effects or benefits which may be as, or even more, important.

Surveys in this field can serve a radical function by providing an alternative to the professional's assessment of the effects of care. This did not happen for all the surveys discussed. The assumption behind

Lorber's studies of the treatment of infants with spina bifida cystica was that the quality of life is, in some situations, more important than survival. Lorber made the assumption on the basis of the observation of an unselected group of treated patients. Zachary rejected the assumption. Neither of them attempted a systematic survey of the viewpoint of the children or parents concerned. In contrast, Shepperdson interviewed the parents of children with Down's syndrome in an attempt to ascertain their views on this issue.

7 Acceptability of services

Concepts of the acceptability of services range from the restricted notion of 'compliance' – the extent to which patients carry out the treatment prescribed by doctors – to the rather wider notion of satisfaction with existing services, and extend to the more radical concept of considering how far services are planned in a way that takes account of patients' experience and preferences. Accessibility is another aspect of acceptability and this in its turn has many facets: geographical, temporal, social and psychological.

In this chapter I cover four services whose acceptability has tended to be assessed in these different ways. So I have looked at compliance over drug taking, accessibility of primary medical care, satisfaction with hospital inpatient care and women's perceptions of childbearing and related services.

Compliance over drug taking

The extent to which it is appropriate to be concerned about patients' compliance with, or adherence to (a pleasanter concept), drug regimens depends on the doctors' therapeutic intentions when prescribing drugs. Some information about this for general practitioners was obtained in a study of 19 doctors in a single town (Logan 1964). These doctors recorded information about all their consultations (totalling 9,405) during two sample weeks. When a drug was prescribed they believed that it would act only as a placebo in 11%, were hopeful of some therapeutic effect or thought this possible in 55%, and a probable one in 24%. Therapy was only specific in 10%. But of course placebos can have a therapeutic effect.

Both doctors' intentions and patients' attitudes towards the drugs are relevant in assessing the effectiveness of the drugs and patients' adherence to the regimens. Patients' expectations about drug prescribing and doctors' perceptions of these expectations have been explored in a number of surveys. Stimson (1976) has described the relationship between the two as a mismatch, since findings suggest that patients expect a prescription at about half the consultations or less whereas the majority of doctors estimate that this happens much more frequently, at around 80% of consultations.

This discrepancy illustrates the value of surveys in correcting perceptions that are almost inevitably based on a biased selection of messages. When patients want prescriptions, it is relatively easy for them to make the doctor aware of this – they can ask directly or hint. It is much less easy to convey a negative wish since it is gratuitous to state that a prescription is not wanted before it is given and it appears to be rejecting the doctor's help to refuse when it is offered. So it is not surprising if doctors get an erroneous impression about this. And the discrepancy between patients' expectations or wishes for a prescription and doctors' perceptions and practices may be widening. Cartwright and Anderson (1981) showed that between 1964 and 1977 the proportion of patients who thought that their doctor was too inclined to give a prescription rose from 2% to 7%. People are probably reluctant to criticise their own doctor, and in 1977, when they were asked about doctors in general, almost half, 46%, thought doctors were too inclined to give prescriptions.

The extent and nature of people's anxieties and scepticisms about taking prescribed drugs, particularly psychotropic ones, is a subject about which there is a lot of illustrative and anecdotal evidence but little hard data. This seems to be a somewhat neglected area. The rejection of prescriptions by not getting them dispensed is one indication of these doubts, but there have been only single area studies of this phenomenon. Without larger, nationally based surveys, we can only speculate about trends over time, the effect of rising prescription charges and the influence of possible changes in attitudes to drugs and to the doctors who prescribe them.

A recent estimate of the proportion of 'uncashed' prescriptions in one area was made in a survey of three general practitioners (Rashid 1982). The doctors were asked to complete a short questionnaire about all the patients seen over a three day period who were given a prescription. The prescriptions 'cashed' were identified at the Prescription Pricing Authority for the area and a comparison revealed a shortfall of nearly 20%. Analyses suggested that patients with diseases that the doctor judged as less severe were less likely to cash prescriptions than those with more serious illnesses, that 'the uncashed prescriptions were often for psychotropic drugs and antibiotics rather than "placebo"-type drugs, such as ascorbic acid and aspirin as might have been expected' and that patients in Social Class IV (semi-skilled occupations) had the highest rate of non-compliance. However it is stated that 'most of the comparisons . . . narrowly missed significance'.

Waters, Gould and Lunn (1976) in an earlier study in a mining practice found a much lower overall proportion of prescriptions that were not made up, 7%, but considerable variation between different types of patients. Among miners aged 25–34 the proportion was 42%.

The extent to which patients are taking drugs that doctors have prescribed for them is a difficult question for surveys to answer directly since patients may be reluctant to admit that they are not doing so. And there is some evidence that surveys of patients over-estimate compliance. For instance Dunnell and Cartwright (1972), although they did not put the question directly to patients but asked those who had been given a prescription during the two weeks before they were interviewed to keep a diary about all the medicines they took in the subsequent two weeks, found that the proportion of medicines not made up or tried was somewhere between 2% and 5% – the higher proportion allowing for a bias among those who did not complete a diary. When asked whether they took their prescribed medicines more, less, or exactly as they had been advised, 80% said they followed the doctor's advice or instructions precisely. Most studies which have estimated compliance in other ways reveal rather higher proportions not adhering to the prescribed regimens. The various methods employed involve checking whether prescriptions are made up, putting a 'marker' in the drug which shows up in the patient's urine or stool, counting the pills that are left over and checking whether patients return for a repeat prescription at an appropriate interval.

Studies that have been based on markers or tablet counting usually have not involved surveys. For instance one study by Porter (1969) on 'drug defaulting' in general practice, used a marker in the urine and residual tablet counting but rejected 'interrogation' as being too subjective. Another study of whether pregnant women took their iron (Bonnar, Goldberg and Smith 1969) verified cooperation in taking oral iron by regular stool tests for iron. They found that after two months 32% were not taking iron tablets and concluded that 'lack of patient co-operation is an important consideration in the treatment and prevention of iron deficiency anaemia of pregnancy'.

But surveys could be incorporated into such studies to explore the reasons for non-compliance, the factors associated with it, and to identify side effects associated with the rejection of drugs.

A survey which estimated compliance in a number of different ways, and looked at one possible reason for non-compliance – lack of comprehension – was carried out in a single practice (Wandless, Mucklow, Smith and Prudham 1979). They attempted to interview all the patients in the practice aged 65 and over 'who were regularly receiving at least one medicine by mouth (excluding short courses of antibiotics) on the day the study began'. These patients were identified from the practice records. Eighty-one, 62%, of these patients were interviewed at home; none of them refused, the others 'could not be found at home on three occasions'. Three measures of compliance were used. The first compliance index, based on the interviewer's assessment, indicated that there was not more than 10% deviation from absolute adherence for 73% of the medicines taken regularly. The second index was based on a tablet count and related the number of tablets estimated to have been taken to the number recommended. It was possible to make this estimate for three-quarters of the drugs. Indices between 90% and 110% inclusive were found for 47%, less than 90% for 45% and over 110% for 8%. The third measure of compliance was based on practice records for the preceding two years. The number of tablets of each medicine which should have been required by each patient receiving constant treatment during that period was compared with the actual number prescribed. Sufficient information was available to calculate this for 82% of the medicines. Indices were between 90% and 110% for 40%, less than 90% for 48% and more than 110% for 12%.

The three measures of compliance were clearly related, but the interviewer's assessments which were based on patients' reports indicated a greater compliance and the authors felt these to be often misleading. Spearman's correlation between the compliance index based on the tablet count and that based on the prescription record was 0.68 ($p < .001$) and the authors estimate that poor compliance with an individual medicine could be predicted accurately in 66% of cases from an analysis of the prescription records, while a combination of prescription record inspection and interview assessment increased the accuracy of the prediction to 86%.

In addition to compliance, the survey also assessed comprehension by relating the daily dose as described by the patient to that recommended by the doctor. 'Despite the fact that only one quarter of the bottle labels had clear instructions and many of these could not be read by the patients, the correct dosage regimen was known for 92% and the correct purpose for 72% of all the medicines taken.' The authors concluded that 'poor comprehension could not therefore be considered responsible for the compliance indices revealed by the tablet counts'.

The survey made no attempt to look at variations in compliance for different types of medicine but it showed that compliance was poorer for medicines taken more than once a day than for those taken just once a day. They found no association between the compliance index based on tablet counts and age, 'mental test score', social class, marital status, living alone, or duration since last contact with the family doctor; but men complied better than women.

A study of deviation from prescribed drug treatment after discharge from hospital (Parkin, Henney, Quirk and Crooks 1976) yielded rather different results in terms of the part played by comprehension or non-comprehension in adherence to drug regimens. This survey covered 130 patients discharged from four hospital wards. Only those with one or more drugs prescribed at the time of discharge, which had to be taken regularly for more than 14 days, were included. The study found that 35% did not have a clear understanding of the regimen and a further 15% understood the prescribed regimen but did not follow the instructions.

An assumption behind all these studies is that compliance matters. This is being increasingly questioned. A leader in the *British Medical Journal* (1979) points out that, for some patients on certain drugs like insulin or clonidine, failure to take them as prescribed can have disasterous effects, but 'correlations between compliance and the effects of treatment have rarely been sought'. One American study which confronted the problem of adherence to drug regimens and the effectiveness of the drugs had such fascinating results that I cannot resist including it. It was essentially a clinical trial of clofibrate, a drug intended to help in the long term treatment of coronary heart disease (Coronary Drug Project Research Group 1980). The authors identified adherence or non-adherence as a pitfall in relation to the assessment of clinical trials because 'there is often a temptation to evaluate the treatments . . . in only the patients who adhered to the treatment regimen'. In this study the physicians assessed adherence by counting or estimating the number of capsules returned by the patient and 'by talking with the patient about possible side effects or problems with the medication, difficulties in remembering to take the capsules and similar topics'. The basic findings are given in Table 4.

In the clofibrate group mortality was significantly lower among the good adherers – but there was a similar difference between good and

Table 4   Mortality rates (in percentages) in patients given clofibrate or placebo by adherence to prescription

Adherence	Treatment Group	
	Clofibrate	Placebo
Less than 80%	24.6% (357)	28.2% (882)
80% or more	15.0% (708)	15.1% (1813)
Total study group	18.2% (1065)	19.4% (2695)

poor adherers in the placebo group! An analysis of the characteristics of good and poor adherers in the two groups could only account for a small portion of the observed differences. The only reasonable explanation seemed to be that there must be characteristics differentiating between good and poor adherers that were not assessed in the project. There was no difference in mortality between good adherers in the clofibrate group and good adherers in the placebo group, but among the poor adherers mortality rates were lower in the clofibrate than in the placebo groups. The authors concluded that no valid conclusions could be drawn from these data.

So compliance, or adherence, certainly matters when it comes to interpreting clinical trials. But the more hardnosed question posed in the *British Medical Journal* leader, 'Is it established that treatment would do more good than harm to those who do not comply?', is a difficult one to answer positively, and can only be attempted in clearly defined and specified circumstances. The data from the Coronary Drug Project Research Group suggest that although those who took their clofibrate were less likely to die than those who rejected it, the difference between the two groups was not necessarily due to the drug. And that study had a clear outcome measure (mortality) and was not concerned with side-effects. For many prescribed drugs the analysis needs to be more complex, taking into account the bad and the good effects. More studies are needed of doctors' intentions and expectations when prescribing drugs. The economic costs of prescribing drugs made up but not taken also need to be assessed.

Accessibility of general practitioner care

Facets of accessibility to this type of care are: proximity to the doctor's surgery, time taken to get there and method of travel, frequency and times of surgeries, waiting time at the surgery, delays in getting an appointment, the willingness of the doctor to visit patients at home, the doctor's availability in emergencies, the willingness and availability of the doctor to consult on the telephone and the doctor's manner and approachability. All these aspects were studied by Ritchie, Jacoby and Bone (1981) for people living in private households. In their national survey they took a sample of people from the electoral register and used special procedures to overcome two problems: the proportion of people who had moved between the compilation of the register and the date of interview; and the number of people aged 16 and over who did not appear on the register because they were ineligible to vote or because they did not return the registration form. The special procedures they used have been described by Blyth and Marchant (1973). Basically this method involves interviewing not only the selected elector, if still living at the stated address, but a sample of any other eligible people there who do not appear on the electoral register at that address.

Ritchie et al identified 5,373 eligible people of whom 89% were interviewed. Information was also obtained from the Family Practitioner Committees or Health Boards about some aspects of the practices of doctors identified by the people interviewed as their general practitioners. Rather surprisingly, perhaps, information was obtained from the patients rather than the FPCs about surgery times and even though patients were only asked about this if they had consulted their doctor in the preceding five years, 22% did not know the times at which morning surgeries began, the time at which evening surgeries ended or whether there was a Saturday surgery. No attempt was made to check the accuracy of the replies that were obtained. The survey showed that 41% of patients attending single-handed practices said the evening surgery ended after 6.30 pm and this proportion declined to 31% of those attending practices with six or more doctors. It would be interesting to know how this related to the ages of the doctors but this information was not obtained even though it would have been possible to get it from the DHSS.

There is a bias in this study resulting from the form of questioning, since people were asked about the last time they consulted their doctor at the surgery. For these consultations they were questioned about appointments, any delays in obtaining an appointment, satisfaction with the time that was fixed and so on. But information was not obtained about a random sample of consultations: people who had few consultations were given the same weight as people who had several.

In addition, if people have a series of clustered consultations for an episode of illness, asking questions about the last consultation will mean that the one at the end of an episode is more often included than one at the beginning or in the middle. Delays, and anxieties about delays, are likely to be greater for consultations at the beginning of an episode.

The way to obtain a random sample of consultations is to ask about all those that took place during a specified period. This has the practical disadvantage of extending, and possible overloading, the interview for those who have had several consultations during that time, while those who did not have any consultations can obviously not be asked any questions about them. To ask about the last consultation may seem a practical alternative but it is not possible to make reliable estimates from such an unrepresentative collection of data.

The assessment of the doctor's availability in emergencies made by Ritchie and her colleagues was based on questions about patients' experience of trying to contact the doctor outside normal surgery hours during the preceding five years. If they had done this more than once, again they were asked about the last time they had tried to do so. Here there is also the problem of a selective bias in what is recalled, due to asking people about events over such a long period: more dramatic occasions may be remembered, more trivial ones forgotten. Selective memory may distance the picture of events that are reported. In addition, the actual question used here illustrates the ambiguity of 'you'; it was: 'In the last five years, have you ever tried to contact your present doctor (or any of the doctors he works with) outside surgery hours, either for yourself or for a member of your family?' Subsequent questions established whether, on the last occasion this happened, it was the informant who needed to see the doctor or some member of his or her family, and whether it was the informant *or someone else* who tried to contact the doctor. Data in the report indicate that 60% of informants had no experience of trying to contact the doctor in the last five years, 20% had tried to contact the doctor, 11% had needed the doctor for himself or herself and someone else had tried to contact the doctor, and in the remaining 9% 'the informant was not directly involved'. In this last group it is stated that 'informants were relating the experience of other people in their family who were registered with their doctor', but the wording of the question does not make it clear whether or not this was intended. I have often wished, when drawing up a questionnaire, that 'thou' was still in common use, as it would then be possible to distinguish between you, an individual, and you, a couple or family. Another approach to assessing the availability of general practitioners was made by a study group for the London Health Planning Consortium – the Acheson report (1981). Practices were sampled in four inner London and four outer London FPCs. This meant that single doctor practices had as much chance of being included as practices with two, three, four or more doctors so that in terms of the service available to patients in the areas the smaller practices had a relatively greater chance of being included. Three time periods were studied: 11 am – 3 pm and 8 pm – 9.30 pm on Mondays to Friday, and Saturday 10 am – 12 pm. Interviewers from the GLC Social Survey Section were instructed to telephone the practice during the allotted time period. Results were classified in this way:

	Code
Spoke to a doctor	1
Spoke to someone other than a doctor who:	
said a doctor was present and available to speak to the patient	2
said no doctor present but gave an alternative number	3
said no doctor present and did not know how patient could contact doctor or said patient could not contact doctor	4
Answering service replied	5
Answering machine/GPO intercept replied	6
Wrong number	7
Number unobtainable	8
Persistently engaged	9
No reply of any sort	0

The report does not give a definition of how often or at what intervals the interviewer should dial before recording 'persistently engaged' nor of how long they held on before classifying it as 'no reply of any sort'. The interviewer did not ring the alternative number (code 3), follow up the information given by the answering machine or service, re-dial a wrong number, or check with the Post Office if the number was unobtainable. Results were presented solely in terms of 'contact' or 'non-contact', codes 1–4 being counted as a contact and 5–0 as a non-contact on the grounds that 'for the patient, the most crucial factor is whether or not it is possible to obtain direct contact with anyone who is in the GP's surgery, even if it is only a reception-ist'. So if the interviewer was in touch with someone who told them that a patient could not contact the general practitioner this was counted as a contact, while if the answering machine or service gave them information about how to get in touch with the general practi-tioner this was classified as a non-contact without further ado! The proportion of responses classified in this apparently rather arbitrary or strange way was not negligible: in the Inner London areas, for 6% of the calls (14% of those analysed as 'contacts') the interviewer con-tacted a person who said there was no general practitioner at the surgery and did not know how he or she could be contacted, while 47% of the calls (84% of the 'non-contacts') were answered by an answering service or machine. The report concludes (page 17) that 'a worryingly large proportion of practices, particularly single-handed practices, could not be contacted at all'. The figures show that the proportions 'contacted' were 40% of single-handed practices com-pared with 49% for other practices in inner London; while for outer London the proportions were, if anything, in the opposite direction, 52% for single-handed, 48% for others. Neither of the differences reached a level of statistical significance at the 5% level and the comment suggests a bias against single-handed practice.

It could be argued that there was a similar bias in a study by Arber and Sawyer (1981). Their survey was carried out in Surrey and south-west London. A table shows clearly that there was no significant difference with type of practice in the proportion of patients who said they could not talk easily to their GP, or in the proportion 'who do not always say everything they want to their doctor'. A third indicator of the ease of communication, the proportion 'saying they do not get enough information', showed a significant difference and the authors conclude: '. . . taking three aspects of communication, we found that there was, if anything, a *better* personal relationship between patients and their doctors as the complexity of the organisation increased'. Again over treatment: '. . . these findings are not statistically signi-ficant but suggest that single-handed doctors may fall down in these respects'. It might be more reasonable to interpret an insignificant difference in this way if other studies, based on a greater number of areas, had shown similar differences. In practice Cartwright and Anderson's (1981) study based on 20 randomly selected areas found no evidence of any trends with size of partnerships, or differences between single-handed doctors and others, in patients' views of their doctors in relation to explaining things to them fully, listening to what they say, taking time and not hurrying them or examining people carefully and thoroughly. (page 17). And Ritchie et al whose study covered a sample of 164 local authority districts found that: 'Most people found their doctor approachable, in that . . . he was easy to talk to and explained things as fully as possible. The proportions who thought otherwise varied very little with the type of practice . . . but rather more with informant's social class and very much more with their age.' Given that Arber and Sawyer's study was confined to two areas in and near London, I think the emphasis they put on their observed, statistically insignificant, differences is unreasonable. Their claim that 'our sample allowed us to compare different types of organisation in general practice because it automatically gave us a representative cross-section of patients who were registered with different types of practices' is misleading; so too is the way that they generalise from their findings from this locally based study.

Yet another study on access to primary care was carried out for the Royal Commission on the National Health Service by the Institute of Community Studies (Royal Commission on the National Health Service 1979). This was carried out in two areas, three wards in Stoke Newington and the Cockermouth-Maryport area of West Cumbria, and aimed to 'concentrate attention on the needs of priority age groups (children and older people aged 69 or more) in poor areas'. In Stoke Newington the sample was selected in two stages: first a sample of people was taken from the electoral register, it having been estimated that the number selected would contain the desired number of people aged 70 or over and parents of a child aged 11 or less. This 'preliminary sample' was then passed to the staff of the Family Practitioner Committee who drew out those patients who fell into the required groups. (This presumably means that children in single parent families had half the chance of being included in the sample as those living with two parents, while parents of large families had exactly the same chance of being included as those with just one child in the age range.) It is stated that 'the aim of this rather laborious process was to preserve the confidentiality of the FPC's records'. In West Cumbria, however, the sample was taken directly from the doctors' list. (The implication is that there was less need to preserve their confidentiality!) Four practices were involved, and it is stated that this meant 'the sample was drawn from nearly all the patients in the area, missing out only one small single-handed practice in Maryport'. Presumably this practice in Maryport refused to take part in the study which is confined to practices who were willing to participate.

Obviously local studies are useful and illuminating for those who are interested in, concerned with or responsible for local services, but I find it puzzling that a Royal Commission on the National Health Service should be concerned with a survey of two small, local areas on what appears to be a biased sample, when more nationally based studies were available. I also find it puzzling that the Department of Health and Social Security should be prepared to fund so many studies on the same subject. The report on the Stoke Newington and Maryport-Cockermouth survey includes 'a cautionary note' to the effect that 'we cannot claim to have nationally representative samples' and points out that they 'looked at the two extremes of the age range missing out the mass of the population'. But the report fails to put the survey within the context of other nationally based studies. There is, for instance, a discussion of 'designated' versus 'open', 'restricted' and 'intermediate' areas but no reference to the extensive work of John Butler and his colleagues in this field (Butler, Bevan and Taylor 1973, Butler and Knight 1975, Butler 1980).

In sum, this seems to be an area which has been widely, but somewhat indiscriminately, surveyed.

Satisfaction with hospital inpatient care

Social surveys in the health field are sometimes equated with studies of patients' satisfaction with their care. In practice, as this review has illustrated, this is only one aspect out of many in the health and health care fields to which surveys contribute. But surveys are the main way of finding out about satisfaction.

Two national surveys of patients' attitudes to hospital care were carried out in 1961 (Cartwright 1964) and 1977–78 (Gregory 1978). Both used the electoral register as a sampling frame, and each finished up with around 750 interviews – but there were many differences in the approach adopted. Cartwright identified her sample by means of a postal screen, while Gregory added some extra questions to the General Household Survey as a trailer to identify hers. The proportion who subsequently proved ineligible was higher from the postal screen (most of these had been in hospital at an earlier time) although the postal screen only asked about in-patient episodes in a particular six month period, while in the interview screen people were questioned about a period of one year. A comparison of the methods used is given in Table 5.

Table 5   Comparison of the methods used in two national studies of inpatient care

	1961 *Cartwright 1964*	1977–78 *Gregory 1978*
Area covered	England & Wales	United Kingdom
Number and type of areas covered	12 parliamentary constituencies	672 wards
Sampling frame for identification screen	Electoral register	Electoral register
Unit identified	Individuals	Addresses
Method of identification of hospital in-patient sample	Postal screen	Interview 'trailer' on GHS
Response rate to screen	87%	Not stated
Period asked about	6 months	12 months
Proportion of those responding positively to screen who were found to be ineligible	15%	4%
Proportion of successful interviews among those identified as eligible	81%	91%*
Age groups covered	21 and over	All ages
Hospital spell asked about – if more than one during study period	Longest	Earliest
Number interviewed	739	768

* Around 5% of the patients identified on the GHS did not agree to a recall and were therefore not included in the sample issued for interview.

In spite of the different methods used, comparisons could usefully have been made between the two studies and it seems surprising that Gregory made no attempt to do this – either in the actual questions asked (although those used in the earlier study were published in an appendix to the report), or in the analysis. For example the time at which patients were woken had different cut off points on the two studies which may make a considerable difference since people are likely to round off to a precise hour or half-hour. Nevertheless, as Table 6 shows, it is clear that there had been some move towards a later waking up time in hospital – although not as great as might have been hoped.

Table 6   Time of awakening on the two studies

Cartwright 1964		Gregory 1978	
	%	%	
Before 5 am	7		
5 am < 5.30	28	12	5.00–5.30
5.30 am < 6 am	27	32	5.31–6.00
6 am < 6.30 am	26	32	6.01–6.30
6.30 am < 7 am	7	16	6.31–7.00
7 am or later	5	6	7.01–7.30
		1	7.31–8.00
		1	after 8.00 am
Number of patients (= 100%)	723	688	Number of patients aged 14 or over = 100%

Certainly, as can be seen from Table 7, the overall proportion of patients who felt they were woken up too early was similar on the two studies. This was because more of those on the later study who were woken after six in the morning regarded it as too early.

A major source of dissatisfaction on both studies was inadequacy of information, but the questions asked were so different that it is not possible to draw any conclusions about trends over time. I discuss this in some detail to illustrate the problems and implications of formulat-

Table 7   Patients' views on waking up times

	Cartwright 1964	Gregory 1978	
	Proportion who found it too early	Proportion who felt it too early	
Before 5.00 am	74%		
5 am < 5.30	68%	67%	5.00–5.30
5.30 < 6 am	45%	47%	5.31–6.00
6 am < 6.30	24%	46%	6.01–6.30
6.30 < 7 am	17%	27%	6.31–7.00
7 am or later	0%	17%	after 7.00 am
All times	44%	43%	All times

ing questions. Cartwright's main question was: 'While you were in hospital were you able to find out all you wanted to know about your condition, your treatment and your progress?', which might be criticised for including condition, treatment and progress all in one question. However the defence would be that people do not always distinguish between them and it is therefore better not to attempt to separate them and more realistic to combine them.

Gregory's first question about information related to eight specific treatments or tests*. For each treatment they had received patients were asked: 'Were you told enough about why it was necessary?' This imposes a limitation on the information that might be wanted as patients could wish to know how it would be done, whether it would hurt, how it might help and so on. Later in the interview Gregory asked a series of more general questions about patients' satisfaction with information starting with: 'While you were in hospital do you think you were always told enough about how you (and the baby) were progressing?' This is limited to progress and there is no question about their satisfaction with the information they were given about their diagnosis, nor about other types of treatment – other than the eight specific ones listed. Cartwright quotes a number of examples of the sort of things patients had wanted to know which do not fall into Gregory's categories.

Another problem about the way Gregory's question is framed is that it seems to assume that patients are initially passive and wait to be told things; they only start asking questions if they are not told anything. Cartwright asked the patients in her survey: 'In general did you ask about things or did people tell you of their own accord?' and reported that 45% said they mainly asked, 40% that they were told, 7% that they neither asked nor were told; 8% did not answer in those terms. Gregory goes on to ask those who did not say they were always told enough: 'Did you feel that you could ask the doctors to tell you what you wanted to know or not?' The assumption here is that doctors were the people from whom patients would seek information. To quote Cartwright's findings again, she found the main source of information was a doctor for 46% of the patients, a sister or nurse for 39%, other

---

* These were: 'a blood sample taken or a blood test; any injections; X-rays; physiotherapy; given a water or urine specimen; a general anaesthetic – (being put to sleep for a short while); stitches or clips or have them removed; dressing done, changed or removed'.

patients for 2%, someone else for 2%. Eleven per cent said no one gave them information.

Gregory classified the answers to her question about feeling able to ask the doctors questions into 'Yes could ask all doctors', 'Yes could ask only some doctors not others' and 'No could not ask any doctors'. This was followed, for those who felt they could ask all or some doctors, by: 'When you asked the doctors what you wanted to know did you generally get a satisfactory answer?' For this in addition to 'Yes' and 'No' there is a classification 'Never asked any questions.' The question as it was framed had assumed that if patients said they did not think they were told enough and that they felt they could ask doctors what they wanted to know, then they would do so. The additional code belies that assumption, but for patients to reply in those terms they had to do two difficult things – they had to reject the question as it was framed, and they had to reveal an apparent illogicality in their actions.

How much difference does the precise form of the questions make? Possibly not much; people may well answer the question they feel should have been asked, and tell the interviewer what they feel is important. Respondents to both Cartwright's and Gregory's question may have been telling the interviewers whether or not they were satisfied with communications while they were in hospital. The proportions responding negatively to the two basic questions were rather different on the two studies: 21% of the patients in Cartwright's survey said they were unable to find out all they wanted to know about their condition, their treatment or their progress while they were in hospital, while 31% of those in Gregory's study did not feel they were told enough about how they were progressing. (An analysis by age suggests that this proportion was somewhat lower for patients aged 21 and over.) Since Gregory's question is theoretically more limited than Cartwright's this suggests a substantial increase in the proportion reporting dissatisfaction. For the sake of a more precise comparison I think it would have been useful if Gregory had asked the same question as Cartwright. I also think Cartwright's question was a better one – but readers must make allowance for an inevitable bias in this judgement!

A series of surveys of patients' views of hospitals has been carried out by Raphael (1969). These were 'not conceived as an academic exercise . . . [but] to evolve, demonstrate and make generally available a practical tool of management'. Essentially the aim was to enable particular hospitals to find out how patients viewed their stay there. Hospitals were invited to participate and there was no intention or aim of covering a random sample of patients in general. Within hospitals, wards were selected for inclusion in the study after discussion with staff members. The ward sisters then gave out questionnaires during the last day or two that patients spent in the ward, together with stamped envelopes addressed to the King's Fund. Patients under 16, those who were in hospital for less than two nights and those who could not read or write in English were excluded. Two methods of returning the questionnaires were tried: in one, patients were asked to return the questionnaires during their last day or two on the ward, in the other soon after they got home. In the experimental trial of these two methods, in matched wards, a rather better response was obtained when patients were asked to return the questionnaires during their last two days in hospital, so this was the method generally adopted for the rest of the study. Raphael also looked at the replies given by the two groups and found what to me was an unexpected result – that those who reported on the hospital after they returned home were less critical than those who answered the questionnaire while they were still in the ward. This held not only for 'overall contentment' but for four out of the five specific topics she analysed. I would have predicted that patients would be more willing to criticise the hospital once they had left it. However, concerning the information they were given, those answering while they were still in hospital were less critical. Raphael speculates that this is because they expected information to be given to them before they left.

The questionnaires were completed anonymously so it was not possible to send reminders. The response rate was 62%. This is comparatively good without a reminder. If the questionnaires had been numbered, it would have been possible to check who had replied and to send reminders to those who had not, but of course it could not have been claimed that the replies were anonymous – merely that confidentiality would be respected and that no individuals would be identified in any report. In my view it would have been useful to do another experiment to ascertain the effect of making the responses anonymous on both the response rates and the nature of the replies. People may be less willing to express criticisms if replies are not anonymous, but we do not know the extent of this effect or even if it exists. On the other hand, it may be the reluctant responders who are more critical, so if reminders were sent and a higher response rate achieved there might be more criticisms. But to send reminders not only means sacrificing anonymity, it also needs careful organisation and clerical resources.

Raphael's questions covered the ward and equipment, sanitary accommodation, meals, activities while in hospital and the care patients were given. Patients were also asked questions which Raphael assesses under a heading of 'overall contentment'. At the end were two open questions at which patients were asked to state what they liked best and what they liked least about their stay in hospital, and there was space for additional comments and suggestions. Nearly all the questions were to be answered yes or no – but there was a space for explanations. Negative responses invariably implied criticism, for example, 'Were your bed and bedding comfortable?', 'Were there enough W.C.s?', 'Did you have enough privacy on the ward?' In my view many of the questions would more appropriately be answered by a scale of intensity or frequency; a yes or no is too simplistic.

Strictly speaking the results from this series of surveys were not additive – it does not make sense to add them since together they do not represent anything that can be defined. It is more appropriate to give results for the individual hospitals included in the study. For the most part Raphael gives both an overall percentage and a range over the different hospitals. Possibly the most fascinating and useful parts of her analyses are those which relate the attitudes of patients in the study hospitals to various attributes of the hospitals, such as cost per in-patient week and catering costs per week, although the former did not relate to patients' 'overall contentment' nor the latter to their comments on the food. She found that 'opportunity for choice of food has a closer relationship to satisfaction with meals than the amount spent on them'.

Raphael included just one question on information: 'Were you told enough about your illness and treatment?'. Unlike Gregory she did not ask about progress but about illness and treatment, but, like Gregory, she put the emphasis on being told rather than on finding out. Altogether 82% of the patients said they were told enough, the percentage varying from 72% to 89% in the ten hospitals participating in the study. This 82% might be compared with the 69% in Gregory's study who said they were told enough about how they were progressing. Some possible reasons for the difference are the nature of the patients included, the response rates, the postal or interview study, the points in time at which the studies were done and the wording of the questions.

Women's perceptions of childbearing and related services

Several studies have looked at women's satisfaction with various aspects of these services. For instance Bone (1973) has looked at satisfaction with different methods of contraception, and with family planning services. Cartwright and Lucas (1974) have considered the acceptability of abortion services to women who had an abortion, while women's views of antenatal care have been studied by O'Brien and Smith (1981), McKinlay (1970), Macintyre (1981), Graham (1978) and others.

Preferences are more difficult to study than satisfactions because they are not usually based on experiences of the possible alternatives. When people are asked which of two forms of care they prefer they tend to favour the one they have experienced. Cartwright (1979), in a survey based on a random sample of births selected from birth certificates, found this was so for women giving birth in home or in hospital, and for women having or not having an epidural but not for women whose birth had been induced. And there are other problems in obtaining meaningful information for women's wishes for a non-existent service. Before the Abortion Act there was apparently no survey of whether women in general, or pregnant women, or women who had had a baby, would have liked the option of an abortion. This may have been for political and financial reasons rather than method-ological ones. If surveys can only usefully study attitudes to existing services, does this mean that they are inevitably a conservative influence – never producing evidence about new services that might be appreciated or suggestions for innovations? I think this is a real danger, but some studies, whose authors might not appreciate them appearing in a section on acceptability, have attempted something rather more ambitious. These have been small-scale, in-depth socio-logical studies of processes and by interpreting their findings and putting them in the context of a body of theoretical, historical and scientific knowledge the authors identify implications for services which are innovative and would tie in with women's preferences and needs.

An example of such a study is Oakley's (1980), which was con-cerned with the process of becoming a mother. She talked to women who were having their first baby, twice in pregnancy and twice in the early post natal months, about 'social and medical aspects of the transition to motherhood'. Her sample was taken from one hospital and restricted to women between 18 and 31, married or co-habiting with the child's father, living within a restricted radius of the hospital and who 'booked in' at the ante natal clinic within the first 25 weeks of their pregnancy. It was a relatively middle class sample: according to their partner's occupation 66% of the 55 who participated throughout were middle class; according to the women's own occupation 93% were.

In addition to the interviews, the majority of which, three-quarters, were done by herself, Oakley had access to the hospital medical notes, she observed six of the births and she made 'extensive observation of obstetric work in the "research" hospital'.

A basic idea behind her study was the suggestion 'that the medicalisation of reproduction has changed the subjective experience of reproduction altogether, making dependence on others instead of dependence on self a condition of the achievement of motherhood' (pages 97–98). At the end she puts forward four proposals for making 'becoming and being a mother a more comfortable experience' (page 1):

'1 An end to unnecessary medical intervention in childbirth.
'2 The re-domestication of birth.
'3 A return to female controlled childbirth.
'4 The provision of therapeutic support for women after childbirth.' (pages 295–296).

Her argument is based on historical, anthropological and ethnomethodological data as well as her survey, but I will focus on the information arising from the survey that is used to support her first and last proposals. Most of the statistical data relate to depression and the associations with various measures.

In assessing 'postnatal depression' Oakley identified four categories: postnatal 'blues', anxiety, depressed mood and depression.

'Each of the four outcomes was assessed on the basis of self-report. . . . For the "blues": "Did you feel at all depressed at any time during your stay in hospital?" For anxiety on homecoming: "What did you feel like when you came home with the baby?" "Did you feel at all anxious about looking after the baby on your own?"

Descriptions of depressed mood could be given at various points in the interview. Each interview also carried the following questions: "How do you feel in yourself apart from the physical side of things?" "Are you suffering with your nerves at all?" "Are you depressed at all at the moment?" Women who said "yes" to questions about feeling depressed or suffering from "nerves" were also asked a series of questions derived from the Present State Examination Schedule, a standardized clinical-type interview developed for the detection of psychiatric morbidity at the Institute of Psychiatry in London. The questions used covered frank feelings of anxiety and/or depression, feelings of tension/inability to relax, undue sensitivity to noise, panic attacks, fear/avoidance of social contacts, self-confidence, concentration, appetite and sleep disturbance, feelings of lethargy and irritability' (pages 115 and 304).

Clearly it was a pretty comprehensive and carefully thought out categorisation. What is not clear from the report on the study is who classified the interview material into the four categories. Apparently it was Oakley herself and there was no independent checking and validation of the categorisation. She has discussed some of the problems she encountered in her interviewing in a thought-provoking paper (Oakley 1981). I think her approach is particularly useful for generating hypotheses and suggesting how they might be explored. It seems less satisfactory or practical for larger-scale studies.

Turning to the analysis, Oakley reports that postnatal blues were related to 'dissatisfaction with second-stage labour', instrumental delivery, and epidural analgesia. Depressed mood was related to 'segregated marital role relationship', housing problems and not being employed; while depression was associated with 'dissatisfaction with birth management', 'medium/high technology score', low control felt in labour and little previous contact with babies. Anxiety was not related to any of these things. Again the categories used are carefully defined in terms of the questions that were asked, or of the data extracted from the medical records.

In the analysis of her findings Oakley discusses the concept of vulnerability and uses a vulnerability index made up of four factors (not being employed, having a segregated marital role relationship, housing problems and little or no previous contact with babies). She did a three-way analysis of high or medium versus low technology, one vulnerability factor against two or more, and depression, and a similar one of depression plus depressed mood. The hypothesis behind the analysis was that 'childbirths that were relatively high in technology "score" would be more potentially stressful maternal experiences and therefore more likely to be followed by depression. Whether or not depression in fact occurred would then be seen as partly a function of social context – being "vulnerable" or "protected" by virtue of the absence or presence of social defences and supports.' (page 174). She showed that all the 13 depressed mothers had both a high or medium technology score and at least two vulnerability factors whereas those with depression or depressed mood, although mainly concentrated in the same group, were found in each of the four groups. And she concludes: '. . . evidently the relevance of the analysis is greater in the case of depression' (page 174).

The discussion is well argued and thought provoking. I have two reservations. The first I have already indicated – an anxiety that with one person generating hypotheses, collecting most of the data, classifying and analysing the data there is an inevitable risk of bias and a clear lack of independence between the different stages. As Macintyre (1980) has put it: 'It appears somewhat ingenuous of [Oakley] to state . . . that the six groups of factors (independent variables) that she had selected and operationalized "*turn out* to be related to outcome" [Macintyre's italics] as if this were a serendipitous finding rather than one at least in part dictated by her preconception of and theorizing about the research, and her selection of questions and factors.' My second reservation relates to the nature of the sample which contained not only a high proportion of middle class women but also seems to have been carried out in a hospital using a lot of technology. This was particularly so in relation to epidural anaesthesia: 79% of Oakley's sample experienced this compared with 10% of the women having first babies in Cartwright's national sample based on births in 1975 (1979 – additional unpublished data). The proportions having an 'instrumental delivery' were 52% in Oakley's sample, 28% of the first births in Cartwright's study, but the induction rates in the two studies were not so dissimilar, and if anything the other way round: 21% in Oakley's study, 26% among the first births in Cartwright's. There was no mention of any Caesarean sections in Oakley's study. So the high technology was not used across the board, but in a way that was atypical. It is obviously well worth identifying some of the disadvantages of such a situation, but of course it is not then possible to generalise from the results to situations in which technology is employed rather differently, and indeed Oakley's study is subtitled 'Towards a sociology of childbirth'. In my view the survey part of her study has generated enough data to suggest that her hypotheses are well worth pursuing with a larger, randomly selected sample in a survey with enough resources to allow the collection, classification and analyses of data to be carried out independently and the classifications checked and validated.

One survey based on large numbers and a quite different type of design was the *British way of birth* (Boyd and Sellers 1982). This was done by asking viewers of a television programme who were at least three months pregnant to take part in a survey on maternity services. Nearly 10,000 letters were received and the authors calculate that almost one woman in every seventy having a baby in Britain responded to the initial request. This could be interpreted as around a 2% participation rate. The women who wrote in were sent a 29 page questionnaire and some 60% returned usable forms. As the authors point out this was 'not a truly statistical survey . . . the women selected themselves . . . this means our survey is biased towards better-educated women . . . 36% . . . were from social class 1 and 2 . . . according to official figures this . . . should have been nearer 25% . . . further only 3% of mothers in the survey were under twenty, while this should have been at least 10%' (page 2). Another bias, not identified in the report, was an under representation of single mothers.

Most of the report on the study is based on quotations and comments of the mothers and reveals many aspects of maternity services that some of them felt were unsatisfactory. The statistical counts are presented in a final chapter which might seem appropriate given the nature of the sample, but I think it would have been helpful to put many of the quotations in the context of the proportion of mothers giving that sort of answer or encountering a problem at that stage. No cross analyses are presented in the report, although such a survey could well show differences between groups and in a subsequent letter to the *British Medical Journal* (Rantzen and Watts 1982) it is shown that 'belt monitors seem to be statistically associated with the sample of "unhealthy" babies, rather than "healthy" ones'.

This type of study has become quite frequent. Claire Rayner in collaboration with the Royal College of General Practitioners recently did a survey among the readers of *Woman's Own* about what they thought of their doctor (1981 and 1982). People responded 'in thousands' and a computer analysis was made of a random sample of replies. A representative of the Royal College was quoted as saying that he hoped 'future training schemes for new general practitioners and continuing education provided for practising general practitioners will take the survey's findings into careful account'. I think such studies can usefully highlight deficiencies in services. I would also hope the general practitioners will take the limitations of the study into account. These relate not only to the 'sample' but also to some of the questions. I do not think much sense can be made of one that asks, 'Will your doctor make home visits – always, never, or sometimes?', although Claire Rayner found the responses to this reassuring.

Another study of maternal attitudes, this time to home confinements, took advantage of a hospital strike to look at mothers' views of unintended home confinements (Goldthorp and Richman 1974). The sample consisted of 65 women, who having been booked for hospital delivery, had their babies at home because of the strike. Asked about their feelings when they had been told that they could not have their baby in hospital as planned, 22% said they felt pleased, 40% did not mind, 20% were disappointed and 18% very disappointed. But after their experience 80% of the mothers wanted to have their next baby at home. The authors recognised that the survey had an obvious bias since it was carried out by local authority midwives who had a vested interest in the continuation of domiciliary deliveries. This study illustrates the usefulness of an opportunistic approach and of taking advantage of an unexpected and unusual situation.

Some other studies of acceptability

The studies I have discussed in this chapter have been concerned with the acceptability of particular services, or of certain aspects of those services. Other services have been looked at from this point of view. Bevan and Draper (1967), Arber and Sawyer (1981) and others have looked at appointment systems in general practice; Clarke (1969) has studied the chiropody service. The home help service has been surveyed by Hunt (1970), dentistry by Gray, Todd, Slack and Bulman (1970), although most of the information obtained from the recipients of these two services was factual and there was little emphasis on their attitudes. Ritchie, Jacoby and Bone (1981) looked at the accessibility of dental, chiropody and ophthalmic services, and of pharmacies, but other aspects of the acceptability of these services do not seem to have received much recent attention. I have discussed some of the surveys of childbearing and related services and their acceptability to women. It is sometimes said that the viewpoint of men about contraceptive services and fatherhood support services is inadequately surveyed. But this situation seems to be changing. Men were included in Cartwright's study of parents and family planning services (1970), in Schofield's (1965 and 1973) and Farrell's (1978) studies of young people, sex and contraception, in Simms and Smith's survey of teenage parents (1982) and in others (McKee and O'Brien 1982). However, surveys have tended to concentrate on married women (Cartwright 1970 and 1979, Oakley 1979 and 1980) and the views of single mothers tend to be overlooked, but with some exceptions (Simms 1982, Macintyre 1977).

The acceptability of health visitor and district nursing services appear to have been surveyed remarkably little. Ritchie, Jacoby and Bone (1981) looked at the accessibility of the services. Many other researchers, even when they have interviewed patients about the help they received from health visitors or district nurses, have not asked direct questions about satisfaction (Hockey 1966, Cartwright, Hockey and Anderson 1973, Cartwright 1970) although some aspect of acceptability has generally been covered, albeit at a limited level.

The acceptability of some types of institutional care has been studied in a variety of ways. Townsend (1962) surveyed residential institutions and homes for the aged, interviewing a sample of new residents, while Carstairs and Morrison (1971) in their survey of the elderly in residential care in Scotland described the standards of accommodation and the staffing of homes but did not attempt to ascertain the views of residents. Others have used ingenious games to try to get at the views of elderly residents who otherwise seemed reluctant or diffident about expressing their wishes for different arrangements (Willcocks, Cook, Ring and Kelleher 1980).

A study of short-stay care of the elderly (Allen 1982) looked at the advantages and disadvantages of short-stay care from the point of view of the elderly people involved, (including those receiving long-term care), their carers and the people organising and running services. It was a sizeable study involving interviews with over 500 people (heads of homes, officers, care staff, long-stay and short-stay residents, carers, social workers, and others involved with the policy and practice of short-stay care), analyses of existing statistics, and postal questionnaires to all social service departments. It aimed to be nationally representative but the sample was biased in two ways: one deliberately, the other not discussed and, apparently, unrecognised. The deliberate bias was to select homes with a high proportion of short-stay admissions. The rationale of this was that 'heads of homes with a lower proportion of short-stay admissions were usually unable to speak authoritatively about the subject'. The unrecognised bias was related to the size of the homes. This was not taken into account either in the initial selection of the homes or in the selection of patients and staff in the homes. This meant that patients and staff from small homes had a greater chance of being included in the study than those in larger homes. If it was intended to interview equal numbers of patients and staff in the study homes then the homes should have been chosen with probability proportional to their size. If the measure of their size had been taken as the number of short-stay residents admitted during a year, then there would have been no need to introduce the deliberate bias and the study would have been based on an appropriate representative sample.

As far as particular aspects of services are concerned, again there seems to be a relative dearth of information about their acceptability. There are few published surveys of patients' reactions to team care in general practice or indeed of health centres – apart from the limited information about these aspects of primary care obtained by Cartwright and Anderson (1981) and the occasional survey in particular practices (Cunningham, Bevan and Floyd 1972, Marsh and Kaim-Caudle 1976). There may be more surveys that look at team care and health centres from the viewpoint of the professionals involved than of the patients.

Turning to procedures, again few surveys have considered the acceptability to patients of alternative methods of treatment. But one study by Jolleys, Barnes and Gear (1978) suggested that the majority of patients preferred endoscopy to barium meal for the investigation of their dyspepsia. However a randomised control trial to compare the result of varicose vein treatment by surgery and by injection/compression schlerotherapy (Beresford et al 1978, Chant, Jones and Weddell 1972) was concerned mainly with clinical outcomes and costs.

Methodological issues

Once again the problems of **single-area studies** arose: two such studies on 'uncashed' prescriptions revealed widely different levels. Another survey of primary health care carried out in only two areas generalised from the findings in an inappropriate way. Only one study of general practitioners' intentions when prescribing drugs has been identified; it covered 19 practices but only a single town.

There were a number of examples of **bias**: the sample design in one study gave patients and staff from small residential homes a greater chance of being included in the study than people in larger homes. Another surveyed self-selected women and was biased towards better educated mothers and away from younger, single ones. A study concerned with access to general practitioner care failed to obtain data about a random sample of consultations as people were asked about the last time they had consulted a doctor. A possible bias was recognised in another study which was carried out by midwives with a vested interest in the results. And interpretations were biased in two studies by putting undue emphasis on insignificant differences which appeared to put single-handed practice in an unfavourable light.

Obtaining accurate data presented difficulties in relation to compliance or adherence to drug regimens. There were also some problems **devising appropriate questions** over information given, or not given to hospital patients, and in making it clear to informants whether 'you' was intended to be single or plural.

The **classification of information** presented some dilemmas. The disadvantages of a single person formulating hypotheses, drawing up the questionnaire, doing the interviewing and analysing the data had to be set alongside the advantages. And a classification of 'contacts' or 'non-contacts' on a telephone study of access to general practice appeared to be arbitrary and somewhat illogical, and led to some misleading conclusions.

There was a somewhat surprising **lack of validation** on a study which accepted patients' statements about their doctor's surgery hours without attempting to check them.

In conclusion

Acceptability has been studied in a limited way for a restricted number of services. Studies of adherence to drug regimens have often

been based on the uncritical assumption that adherence is a good thing
and there does not appear to have been any study relating adherence to
the doctors' intentions and expectations when prescribing drugs.
Occasionally, an excessive number of surveys seem to have been
carried out in one particular field. But in general there are a wide range
of services, treatments and procedures over which we are ignorant of
users' and potential users' attitudes and preferences. Parents' and
children's views of the school health and other child care services, and
the attitudes and experiences of patients who have used emergency
ambulance services are two services where there seems to be little or
no information. Diagnostic procedures often develop apparently
without any survey of which procedure is more acceptable to patients
or of whether, from the patients' viewpoint, the knowledge gained is
worth the discomfort and tribulations involved in obtaining it. Treatments too are assessed without an input of patients' feelings and
experience. Why has the feminist movement not insisted on studies of
consumer reactions to early abortions performed by dilation and
curretage and by vacuum aspiration?

In the past it was probably accepted that professionals were the
most appropriate, indeed the only relevant, judges of what investigations and treatments should be carried out. And the organisation of
services was determined by economic and political considerations.
Now we have a National Health Service, a consumer movement with
at least some recognition of its role in the service, and a public that is
increasingly interested in and informed about health, it is surprising
that surveys of acceptability are not carried out more generally, and
taken into greater account when planning services and determining
appropriate treatments and investigations.

One reason why this may not have been done more often is that
patients tended to say they were satisfied whatever the circumstances.
We are now probably more skilful at eliciting criticisms and reservations and patients are almost certainly more willing to express them.
Another reason for an earlier reluctance to carry out such studies was
the disapproval of the medical establishment. I recall the initial
disbelief followed by horror with which the General Medical Services
Committee reacted in 1963 when informed that I was planning to ask
patients what they thought about their general practitioners. Thirteen
years later, when we wanted to do a similar survey, they were much
more relaxed about it. And a number of doctors are carrying out
surveys in this field – for example the studies by Devlin, Plant and

Griffin (1971) on surgery for anorectal cancer and by Beer and his colleagues (1974) on ambulances to physiotherapy which I quoted in the previous chapter. I hope more such surveys will be done in the future.

8 *The organisation of health care*

The ways in which surveys have illuminated this area are complex and varied. I have looked mainly at studies in three broad categories: first, international comparative surveys which consider the way different organisational systems work out in practice; second, surveys concerned with variations in health care and the organisational factors associated with these variations; and third, surveys from the perspective of health professionals.

International comparative studies

Within a country such as ours with a National Health Service the scope for studying the implications of basically different forms of health service organisation is limited, and international comparisons are appealing. However if we are to compare the output of services in terms of use and satisfactions we also need to know whether levels of need are similar or the extent to which they differ.

A study of health and health care on an international collaborative basis was carried out in 1968/69 (Kohn and White 1976). This was a mammoth undertaking, based in twelve centres and seven countries. Interview questionnaires were administered to 47,648 individual respondents. The study was 'concerned with the extent to which personal determinants of health and health behaviour such as psychological, biological and social factors affect the use of health services, and how these relationships are modified by selected characteristics of the prevailing health services systems' (page 1). Methodologically, 'none of the areas under study represents national or regional populations, nor are the services used to be taken as representative of national or regional systems' (page 7).

However it was felt that the study 'should provide opportunities for achieving new insights into health care processes and health services systems, with the general objective of improving them' (page 7). 'As pieces of information are collected from a wide variety of macrosystems in different places and countries, it should be possible for the World Health Organization to accelerate understanding of medical care processes as well as of the structure and functioning of health services systems' (page 7).

Household surveys were carried out in the twelve study areas, eight different sampling schemes being adopted because of the varying sampling frames that were available. Response rates from eligible individuals ranged from 89.8% to 99.9% in the twelve areas – a staggering achievement since there were 307 questionnaire items for adults and 236 for children. These covered use of services, perceived morbidity, psychobiological dysfunction, health related attitudes, family financial resources and accessibility of medical care along with demographic characteristics.

A great many data have been systematically collected and analysed and the participants in the study learnt much about their own and other countries, about methodological problems in carrying out surveys and about organisational problems in conducting studies in different countries. But it is difficult to draw policy implications from this mass of information. Under their final heading, 'Implications for health care policy', the authors make no clear policy recommendations arising from the study, but point out the need for the 'continuous monitoring of the efficacy, effectiveness and efficiency of all health services and the importance of distinguishing between preventive, counseling, curing and caring functions' (page 399). However they do quantify the variations in perceived needs, resources and use of services in the twelve areas, and they discuss the implications of these variations. A summary of one of their 'major findings' illustrates, to my mind, the extent and the limitations of this type of approach.

'Referrals by physicians showed a more than four-fold difference among the study areas and tended to be more frequent in all five European study areas, probably reflecting differences between the relatively unstructured systems in the six North American study areas and Buenos Aires and the more structured systems in the five European study areas. This is consistent with the finding that the latter study areas tended to have fewer systems points of entry than the other study areas; Helsinki was the exception' (page 394).

The technical and organisational achievement of the Kohn and White study can be better appreciated when it is compared with a **qualitative survey of health, health services and housing in eight member countries of the European Communities** – 1977 (Statistical Office of the European Communities 1981). In this study representative surveys of the eight countries were attempted, the intention being to 'use some form of probability sampling based on comprehensive and up-to-date registers' (page 50). In practice, France mainly used a quota sampling method, in Belgium individuals within selected households were not interviewed on any systematic or appropriate basis, in Italy 'communi' were chosen on the basis of whether they were in a position to carry out the survey successfully, while in the Netherlands 32% of the sample were not contacted, this proportion rising to 40% in municipalities and 65% in the three largest towns. Among those contacted the response rate was poor in Germany (65%) and relatively low in Ireland (74%). Another problem was that substitutes were taken in both Italy and the Netherlands. So only Denmark and the UK adhered to an appropriate sample design and obtained a reasonable response.

Questions on health services related to both use and satisfactions. The proportion who had consulted a doctor in the previous twelve months varied from 57% in Ireland to 76% in France (UK 70%) while the proportion who had been in hospital during that time was considerably higher in France, 21%, than in the other countries, between 8% and 12% (UK 9%). Dissatisfactions with health services were much greater in Italy where 27% were fairly or very dissatisfied compared with between 3% and 16% in other countries (UK 7%). Questions on health asked about people's satisfactions with their health, the presence of specific symptoms in the previous four weeks and ability to do certain day-to-day things. People in France and Italy reported the most symptoms, those in Belgium and Ireland the least.

This survey was essentially an experimental one 'to test the extent to which the concepts and questions used in such a survey could usefully cross cultural and linguistic frontiers' (page 1), but it was also designed to provide information required by the Communities.

A different type of **comparative study of health systems and medical care was carried out in two institutions for the elderly**, one in Scotland – Scottsdale; the other in California – Pacific Manor (Kayser-Jones 1981). The two institutions were selected as being representative of the type of institution that provided medical services and nursing care for the elderly with chronic physical disabilities. Both had a good reputation locally since one of the aims of the study was 'the identification of institutional structures that contribute to high quality care' (page 10). Scottsdale was under the National Health Service, while Pacific Manor was a proprietary nursing home which admitted only privately funded patients, although half the patients were on Medicaid at the time of the study since they had used all their savings to pay their bills and were by then on welfare (page 66). Both participant observation and formal interviews were used to gather the data. The formal interviews showed that patients in Scottsdale were much more satisfied with their care than those in Pacific Manor and the observational studies indicated that this reflected real differences in the quality of the care they received. Kayser-Jones identified three problems at Pacific Manor which contributed to the lower quality of care there:

'1 a lack of leadership and responsibility by professionals (doctors and registered nurses) for the care of the aged

'2 accountability for care at Pacific Manor is not to health professionals, it is to the proprietor of the institution who hopes to make a profit and who is in turn accountable to the State Department of Health to avoid being closed for violations of regulations, and

'3 the organisation and financing of health care contributes to the pauperization and stigmatization of the aged' (page 121).

She found that 'The withdrawal, depression, loss of hope, and desire to die expressed by patients at Pacific Manor had no analogue at Scottsdale.'

Her conclusions support the value of a National Health Service and of the teaching of geriatrics in medical schools. But as Sir George Godber pointed out (1981) there are many units in Britain which fall far short of the standards in Scottsdale. There are other problems in the interpretation of the data: expectations of patients may be different; those receiving care under the National Health Service may be less willing to criticise their care than privately funded patients. The comparison highlights the deficiencies of the American system but certainly should not be used to bolster complacency here. A basic problem is that one of the techniques adopted on this study – that of participant observation – is not appropriate for large scale studies, and that more broadly based studies are needed to support the conclusions.

Another **cross national study of elderly people** was carried out in three countries: Britain, the United States and Denmark (Shanas et al 1968). This was based on structured interviews with national samples of approximately 2,500 persons aged 65 and over living in private households in each country. Response rates among the identified individuals varied from 84% to 90%. The broad aim was to show to what degree old people, in different ways, are integrated in industrial society. Some of the findings related to health and health services were:

1 'Old people in the United States are less likely than old people in either Denmark or Britain to be housebound or restricted in their mobility or to report incapacities in functioning' (page 46).
2 'In Britain the elderly receive slightly more medical consultations; more of them are visited by a doctor when ill in bed at home; more of the housebound and of the bedfast are visited regularly by a doctor' (page 97).
3 'In the United States there is greater emphasis on, first, hospitalization, second, short stays in hospital, and, third, treatment in a clinic, office, or surgery, than in the two European countries' (page 97).
4 'Over a range of everyday personal and household tasks – for example, housework, meals, shopping, bathing and dressing – the great majority of those old people who experience difficulty rely on husbands and wives, children and other relatives for assistance' (page 429).
5 '. . . among the older age-groups (75 or more) relatively more old people in Britain and (though to a lesser extent) in Denmark than in the United States report impairments . . . Paradoxically the incapacitated in Britain more often say their health is good than in either of the other two countries' (page 445).

The last finding illustrates the danger of just taking people's perception of their health as an index.

A comparative study of professionals was carried out by Mechanic (1972) who looked at the work of primary care physicians in the United States and in England and Wales. He compared his sample of general practitioners in England and Wales (Mechanic 1968 – discussed later in this chapter under professional preferences) with a sample of office based general practitioners, internists, pediatricians and obstetricians selected with the help of the American Medical Association. In different medical systems it is difficult to know what are appropriate comparisons. For example, Mechanic was uncertain whether or not to include obstetricians but did so on the grounds that British general practitioners do a considerable amount of obstetrics. He made five approaches to the American doctors and obtained a 66%

response. He found that British general practitioners saw many more patients in their surgeries and on home visits.

American primary care physicians used a wider array of diagnostic procedures, were more closely associated with professional colleagues and expressed less frustration and dissatisfaction. Mechanic points out that his data are descriptive rather than evaluative and implications for public policy do not naturally flow from them but 'when viewed in a larger context these data provide some appreciation of the advantages and difficulties of primary care practice in the two countries'.

A sixth international comparative study is different again. Titmuss (1970) looked at the **scientific, social, economic and ethical issues involved in the procurement of human blood**. His main comparisons were between England and Wales and the USA but he also drew on data from the Soviet Union, South Africa and other countries. In his analysis, Titmuss used available statistics, some earlier surveys and also instigated a survey of donors in England and Wales in 1967. Unlike the other comparative studies I have discussed his did not attempt simultaneous, comparable surveys in different countries. His conclusions are clear and have straightforward policy implications:

> 'On four testable non-ethical criteria the commercialised blood market is bad. In terms of economic efficiency it is highly wasteful of blood; shortages, chronic and acute, characterize the demand and supply position and make illusory the concept of equilibrium. It is administratively inefficient and results in more bureaucratization and much greater administrative, accounting and computer overheads. In terms of price per unit of blood to the patient (or consumer) it is a system which is five to fifteen times more costly than the voluntary system in Britain. And, finally, in terms of quality, commercial markets are much more likely to distribute contaminated blood; the risks for the patient of disease and death are substantially greater. Freedom from disability is inseparable from altruism' (page 246).

But surveys contributed little or nothing to these conclusions. The study in England and Wales provided a picture of the age, sex, social class, marital status, employment, income group and motivation of the blood donors there. Comparisons were made of the basic demographic characteristics of donors and the general population but a comparison of their attitudes with those of a sample of the general population would, in my view, have made interpretation less speculative. Whether it would have strengthened Titmuss's argument is less certain.

My assessment of the appropriate role of international comparative studies is that to illuminate policy they need to be addressed to specific and clearly defined issues. Under those circumstances they can make a substantial contribution to the understanding of the implication of organisational policies. But the main beneficiaries of the more general, broader based cross-national studies are those involved in initiating and setting up the research; for them the experience is likely to be stimulating and educative.

Variations in care

Most of the studies in this field start from one of three perspectives: variations between geographical areas, variations in professional practices and variations with social class in the experiences of patients. In practice the three types of variation are often strongly related, but I shall consider them under the three headings.

Geographical variations In this category I have looked at a series of studies concerned with the prescribing of drugs by general practitioners. This has wide area variations which do not appear to be related to such simple things as the age structure of the population covered. One of the earlier studies that identified this problem was carried out by Martin (1957). His study (not a survey) was based on an analysis of prescriptions in 67 county boroughs with populations between 50,000 and 300,000. He related the data from the prescriptions to information about the doctors' practices obtained from the Ministry of Health, and to data about the areas and their populations. He found that 'all the methods of analysis stress the importance of "custom" and demonstrate the long-standing between-area pattern of prescribing habits'. And he concluded: '. . . one could probably get as good a prediction of the average frequency of prescription per patient in 1951 by using the comparable figures for 1933 as by using any amount of contemporary information' (page 108).

The problem was approached in a number of ways by a group of workers at the Social Medicine Research Unit at the London Hospital in the sixties. Lee, Draper and Weatherall (1965), with no reference to Martin, carried out a survey in three towns which had, over the years, prescribing rates that were markedly different. The study started with an analysis of the statistics available, both for the three towns and the single-handed doctors within them. From this analysis they concluded that 'the main influence on a doctor's prescribing is the town in which he works and that little if any demonstrable differences can be referred to the medical school in which he was trained'. They found no significant relationships between prescribing and the use of home nursing or casualty departments. They went on to interview a random sample of the doctors in the three towns, and 'collected information about their views on many aspects of general practice, the National Health Service and medicine to-day'. In an analysis of these data Joyce, Last and Weatherall (1968) conclude that 'the principal reasons for the differences in prescribing habits between towns are still elusive'. However, by an elaborate and essentially unrepeatable condensing of much of their material by four judges into 16 qualitative scales and a multivariate analysis of the scales, they identified three factors which they tentatively labelled 'quality of practice', 'whole person orientation' and 'education'. They estimated that not more than 15% of the variation in individual patterns of prescribing could have been accounted for by the personal factors studied. Their final conclusion was that 'in general, higher educational qualifications and an orientation towards the whole person were associated with lower prescribing of drugs of all kinds'. In this paper they refer to Martin's work showing the wide variations in prescribing between towns but make no reference to his findings.

The next group to tackle this problem on any scale was the Medical Sociology Research Centre at Swansea (Parish, Stimson, Mapes and Cleary 1976). They studied 859 doctors who went into general practice in England and Wales during a twelve month period 1969/1970. In deciding to approach the problem in this way they apparently underestimated the administrative difficulties for the research posed by the mobility of doctors in the early part of their careers (Webb and Williams 1972). In their main study, response rates to postal questionnaires sent six months after the doctors entered practice, and then between two and two and a half years later, were 64% and 63% of the doctors identified as still being in practice at that time. No analysis of the characteristics available from the Department of Health and Social Security of the doctors who failed to respond is referred to, even though prescribing data would presumably be available for some of them. But because of 'many difficulties in extracting the prescribing data in a usable form' from the Prescription Pricing Authorities, most of the analysed data on prescribing relate to 'a sample of 116 cohort doctors' prescriptions' for one month each between June 1970 and November 1971. So there is the added problem of seasonal fluctuations in prescribing rates and costs. Since the doctors' views and practices could not be related to characteristics of their patients, nor, in the analyses of their prescribing repertoires (Parish and Austin 1976), were they related to prescribing rates or numbers of patients, it is not surprising that few explanatory findings emerged from this large study (86,498 prescriptions issued by the 116 doctors were analysed). Indeed, if the findings from the earlier studies are accepted, studies of new entrants are less likely to reveal large differences between doctors since it may take them some time to adjust to and accept the customs of an area. Presumably the study design arose from an intention to study the socialisation process and the changes in the prescribing of the cohort doctors over time. In practice I have not been able to trace any paper or reference in which such analyses were carried out. It would appear that the project was discontinued before these were done. So the variations persist and surprisingly little has emerged from the surveys to illuminate them.

Variations in practices In **general practice** the main organisational variables to which actions or practices have been related are number of partners, employment of ancillary staff, health centre versus non health centre practice, equipment available, appointment systems, use of deputising services and size of list. The actions that have been related to these organisation variables have included referrals, prescribing, performance of certain clinical procedures, use of various diagnostic procedures, and carrying out of preventive measures.

One study which looked at another aspect of variations in practice was concerned with the **management of hypertension**. It was reported in two parts (Fulton et al 1979; Parkin et al 1979). An opinion survey was carried out in one health board area. All the general practitioners in the area were sent a postal questionnaire and 74% replied. They were asked about the way they measured blood pressure and the place of care, investigation and treatment under certain circumstances. There was general agreement on the type of patient they would refer to hospital and on a diuretic as the drug of first choice in the treatment of mild hypertension, but differences of opinion on the level of diastolic blood pressure at which they would start treatment, the number and type of investigations and the frequency of follow up visits. The more recently qualified doctors proposed rather more investigation and they suggested fewer referrals to hospital. The level of blood pressure at which doctors were prepared to start treatment was influenced by the presence of symptoms although the authors point out it has been shown that symptoms are seldom directly attributable to hypertension

It is stated in the discussion that certain attitudes appear to be related to the size of partnership; from the text it seems that these attitudes related to informing patients about risks of hypertension and the likely need for treatment to continue indefinitely, to support of screening programmes, to use of a nurse in diagnosis and treatment and to the way blood pressure was measured. But no figures are presented about these relationships and there is no attempt to separate the effects of year of qualification and number of doctors in the partnership, although it is recognised that the two go together.

The second part of the study was based on some of the doctors who participated in the first part, but not a randomly selected group. The reason for this is not stated. Each of the 71 doctors who took part in this stage were asked to list five patients whom they considered to have hypertension and who attended the surgery for any reason after a specific date. Data about these patients and their management were then extracted from the practice records.

In over one third of the records only one blood pressure had been entered before beginning treatment. The authors quote Hart (1975) as considering that three blood pressure readings are essential before the diagnosis can be confirmed and as having shown (Hart 1970) that a single reading leads to a misleadingly high prevalence. It would seem that between 7% and 18% (the figures are presented graphically in such a way that a more precise estimate cannot be made) of the patients had the four investigations recommended in an editorial of the Journal of the Royal College of General Practitioners (1976). The way the data are presented make it impossible to say how many were followed up at least once every three months as recommended: it is only possible to say that not more than 2% had three or more blood pressure readings, all the recommended tests and were followed up within the three months.

Some other findings show that a third of the patients were referred to hospital, that men were more often referred than women and that among those looked after by the general practitioner men had more investigations than women. There was no significant difference in the initial blood pressure levels between men and women, but initial levels were higher among those referred to hospital than among those cared for by the general practitioner. No analyses by organisational characteristics are presented in this second paper. There was no difference between general practitioner cases and hospital referrals in the latest blood pressure recorded. The authors conclude that: '. . . the general practitioner is willing to care for the majority of patients himself, to undertake a certain amount of investigation, and to use up-to-date therapy. The result of his treatment in terms of the latest blood pressure is comparable with that of the hospital'. The interpretation seems to me to portray general practitioner care in a good light and to ignore some of the less favourable findings. At the same time I think the authors are to be congratulated for their courage in venturing into this field which not only identifies variations in practices but puts them alongside recommended criteria.

Turning to **hospital practice** there have been relatively few surveys relating organisational aspects of the service to practices. For example I have not found any studies showing whether and how practices vary with the proportion of time consultants spend working for the NHS or with their merit awards. Nor have there been many studies looking at variation in practices with the rank of the doctor.

One study looked at case fatality of hyperplasia of the prostate in two teaching and three regional-board hospitals (Ashley, Howlett and Morris 1971). Patients were interviewed within a week of admission, again in the out-patient department three to six months after discharge and in their own homes about a year later. An abstract was made of data in the case notes and patients were routinely monitored by the Office of Population Censuses and Surveys. The study showed negligible variations between the hospitals in the fatality rate among the planned admissions, but the proportion of unplanned admissions varied from 19% to 82% in the five hospitals and among these emergencies there were wide variations between the hospitals in the proportion operated on. Non-operation carried a high mortality rate and the teaching hospitals operated on a greater proportion of the unplanned admissions – with considerable success.

The authors concluded that: '. . . some regional-board hospitals have to carry a greater burden than teaching hospitals, different services are required of them, and they have to work under greater pressure. Yet, as far as resources are concerned, they are the poor relations.' They went on to comment on 'the loose – even random – matching of needs and resources in the medical and social services'.

And they concluded: 'For a start nobody seemed to have the facts.' They were unable to replicate the main features of their study on a national scale because they could not overcome 'the basic defect of the Hospital In-patient Enquiry – that it deals in admissions, not persons'. Twelve years later this defect and the dearth of data in this field persist.

An unpublished finding from that study was that people who had been operated on by junior doctors took longer to get back to work than those whose operation had been done by a consultant. It seemed that the doctor doing the operation usually did the follow up, too, and junior staff took longer to discharge patients (Ashley, personal communication).

Variations in the experiences of patients The main source of survey data on inequalities in health care is the General Household Survey which was described and discussed in an earlier chapter. Nearly all the data on this topic are derived from studies which were not focused directly on inequalities but which included information on social class or income or education and carried out analyses revealing inequalities. Such studies relate to the use of preventive services, the acquisition of information, and delay in seeking care. One finding from a number of studies is that working class people differ little from middle class in their desire for information but the middle class are more successful in obtaining it (Earthrowl and Stacey 1977, Cartwright 1979).

Surveys have also thrown light on some of the mechanisms contributing to inequalities, and the differential use of services. A number of these are discussed in an article by Cartwright and O'Brien (1976). They include surveys of knowledge and education, of attitudes, self confidence and diffidence, of vulnerability and of the nature of general practitioner consultations.

Hart (1971) discussing the uneven distribution of care and its historical background, summed up the findings in the 'inverse care law – the availability of good medical care tends to vary inversely with the need for it in the population served.' A number of the mechanisms he identified as contributing to this relate to the perspective of professionals. Surveys about this are discussed next.

The perspectives of health professionals

Surveys of the experiences and viewpoints of health professionals are relevant to the organisation of health care in a number of ways. There are analyses of how they spend their time, and the way this varies with different forms of organisation. There are studies of their training and experience, and how these are related to their competence and interest in certain fields of health care. Professional preferences for particular forms of organisation as well as their career preferences may influence the structure of services and will affect the distribution of professionals, while surveys of particular professional groups may have a bearing on the way these groups are utilised.

Analyses of work and time spent on different activities These types of study are more common among nurses than among doctors, but there is at least one observational study of general practitioners and there have been some studies of the hours worked by junior hospital doctors.

A national survey of **community nurses** (Dunnell and Dobbs 1982) aimed first to provide a profile of nurses working in the community – their training, experience, and qualifications; secondly, to produce an outline of their activities related to the client groups being cared for; and thirdly, to relate patterns of work within health districts to the characteristics of those districts.

The study was carried out in 24 out of a sample of 25 systematically selected health districts. In each area the aim was to include half the district nurses, all the other nurses working in the community and employed by health districts, and those employed by general practitioners. Eighty-nine per cent of the general practitioners in the study areas cooperated by identifying their practice nurses and 95% of the nurses identified took part in the study, which involved an interview and keeping a diary about their work activities for seven days.

The study illuminates a wide range of interests. For instance, comparing attached and non-attached district nurses and health visitors it shows greater satisfaction among the attached in terms of opportunity to discuss patients with doctors but no difference in the proportion of time spent in travel or with patients. Eighteen per cent of health visitors have family planning certificates compared with 26% of midwives. Similar proportions of the two had attended management courses in their current jobs, but 78% of the midwives against 42% of the health visitors had been on refresher courses during this time. The length of time they had worked in the community was similar. The midwives spent a rather higher proportion of their time travelling than did the health visitors, but the midwives also spent more time with patients, the health visitors spending nearly half their time on 'non-clinical activities' – mainly clerical and administrative work. Looking at the qualifications of the district nurses, the higher their qualifications the less time they spent in patients' homes. Variations between districts are also reviewed. This survey provides basic data for planning and organising a service. Sometimes attempts are made to collect such information on a routine basis. This often results in vast quantities of inadequate data and much frustration among both those providing the information and those attempting to use it. Ad hoc surveys seem to be a much cheaper and more effective way of obtaining reliable data which are likely to be analysed and used.

A study, which strictly falls outside my definition of a survey because it was based solely on observations, looked at the time spent by **general practitioners** on various professional activities (Buchan and Richardson 1973). As they explain, 'the nature of the study was such as to make selection of general practitioners essential chiefly on the grounds of their expected co-operation' (page 11). They approached 25 doctors whom they estimated would give some degree of representativeness in terms of age, type of practice and list size. Three of those approached declined to take part. The others were observed during six sessions by 'a young doctor doing research' who classified their activities into such categories as history, examination, treatment, advice/reassurance, writing, filing, telephoning, meeting colleagues, and timed how long was spent on each. The study aimed to examine the effect on length and content of consultations of a) the patient's illness, age and social class and b) the doctor's age, practice location, type and list size.

Some of the many fascinating results from that study were:

1 The average 'face to face' time for a consultation was 5.0 minutes at the surgery, 5.6 for home visits.
2 Travel to home visits took 4.7 minutes on average.
3 Two per cent of surgery consultation time was spent on writing certificates. The authors comment that in view of the 'nuisance' value doctors attribute to this task, this is perhaps an example of how the nature of a task can distort perception of time.
4 The number of patients per doctor showed no correlation with face-to-face consulting time.
5 'There was, however, a weak correlation between the average number of patients seen per surgery and the proportion of patients

who were discharged, suggesting that under pressure doctors are less likely to initiate return consultations' (page 17).

6 The average 'face-to-face' time declined from 6.1 minutes for patients in Social Class I to 4.4 in Social Class V. This trend was not noticeable among the patients of rural doctors and could not be explained by differences in illness patterns or in the ages of the patients.

It would have been useful if this study had been extended to include interviews with the patients to ascertain whether patients could make reliable estimates of the time they spent with the doctor, and if the amount of time spent was associated with satisfaction with different aspects of care.

I find it somewhat surprising that this type of study has not been repeated elsewhere or at other times. One problem in carrying out such inquiries is the willingness of doctors to participate. An approach to a random sample of general practitioners asking them if they were willing to participate in a study which involved tape recording of two consultations (if the patients were willing) and agreeing to patients being approached for interviews before and after a consultation led to 18% agreement (Cartwright, Lucas, O'Brien 1976). That study found that the average conversation time was greater at consultations with middle class patients than with working class (Cartwright and O'Brien, 1976).

A survey of **junior doctors'** workload was carried out by the BMA and reported briefly in the *British Medical Journal* (1980). The survey covered 1641 junior medical staff from housemen to senior registrars in NHS hospitals in London and the north-west. It is stated that there was a disappointing response but no further details are given! The main emphasis of the survey seems to have been on pay. Poor response rates seem to be obtained from this professional group. In 1975, a survey of junior hospital doctors' and dentists' hours of duty was carried out for the Review Body on Doctors' and Dentists' Remuneration (Department of Health and Social Security 1975). Only 15.3% of those in full-time work returned usable forms. Comparisons with the proportion claiming extra duty allowance (given in the supplement to the fifth report) suggested that the response was greater among those working longer hours. In its main report the review body states: 'Overall, full-time staff covered by the survey reported their weekly hours of duty as being 85.6 on average, of which 43.2 were normal duty hours and 42.4 were spent on stand-by or call outside these hours.'

Training and experience While there have been several studies of students' and doctors' career preferences, surveys appear to have been relatively little used in attempts to evaluate the training of professionals. The Royal Commission on Medical Education 1965–68 (1968) commented: 'We have had to accept, for our purposes, the virtual absence of systematic factual information about the practical processes of medical teaching in Britain and their effectiveness; we have recommended that provision be made for proper study of the aims and methods of medical teachers as part of a substantial research effort in medical education in coming years' (page 20). At their instigation a survey of first year and final year medical students in 1966 was carried out by the Association for the Study of Medical Education. Response rates were 96% and 95%. The study covered previous education, parental occupation, students' living arrangements, travelling time, participation in various college activities, career preferences and any doubts about their choice of medicine as a career. Final year students were also asked about their course and their reactions to it. Some of the most widely quoted results relate to social class. When students were classified on the basis of their father's occupation, 40% of first year students were in Social Class I compared with 3% of the economically active population in the 1961 census. For those at Oxford and Cambridge the proportion was 51%. Twenty-one per cent of the first year students had medical fathers. Thirty-one per cent of the students in English and Welsh medical schools had been to independent secondary schools. Final year medical students were more likely to express doubts about their choice of medicine as a career than were those in their first year.

One imaginative and unusual study was initiated by a group of clinical students who felt that the problems related to **family planning** were inadequately covered in their clinical course (Simpson 1969). The British Medical Students Association attempted to carry out a survey of final year students at all medical schools in Great Britain to discover what teaching the students had received in that field and their opinions about it. The questionnaires were distributed through BMSA representatives in the medical schools who addressed the envelopes and kept a record of the names and serial numbers on the questionnaires. The questionnaires were returned individually directly to the BMSA in London in pre-paid envelopes. Two reminders were sent to those who had not replied. Four medical schools did not participate and there were some problems in identifying the numbers to whom questionnaires had been sent at some of the other schools, but in the schools that took part in the study the response rate was around 70%. Unfortunately, because of time constraints on the students organising the study, no pilot was carried out and one or two of the questions were misunderstood.

Results showed that 16% of the students who filled in the questionnaire said they had had no teaching in contraceptive methods, and less than half of those who had been taught had had any contact with patients over this. Over a third of all students felt their knowledge of contraceptive techniques professionally inadequate. Teaching in normal psycho-sexual development, marital adjustment and sexual difficulties unrelated to marriage was regarded as even less adequate; only between one-fifth and three-fifths of the students had received any teaching in these fields and less than two-fifths felt their knowledge adequate on any of these three subjects. Nearly all the students, 97%, had received some teaching on infertility and 73% thought their knowledge was professionally adequate. Differences between the medical schools were presented.

A study which looked at the experience of **doctors going into general practice** for the first time was carried out by the Department of Health and Social Security (1972). The aim was to find how far their previous medical experience was relevant to their future needs. Fewer assistants responded, 67%, than unrestricted principals, 82%, but it was thought that this could be explained by the relatively short time they remained in their posts and the consequent difficulty in locating them. It concluded: '. . . few of the new entrants had the experience considered necessary by the Royal Commission . . . there is little evidence of a planned approach to training, the implication being that advice, if available, was not taken, that suitable training programmes did not exist, or that there had been no initial intention of pursuing a career in general practice' (page 22).

Since then vocational training schemes for general practice have become mandatory and the concern is now to evaluate their effectiveness. So far few surveys have been done in this field. Freeman and Byrne (1976 and 1977) made assessments which involved tests and have shown improvements in 'clinical factual recall' and 'problem-solving skill in patient management'. Their findings on any changes in attitudes have yet to be published. Work is in hand to examine whether these improvements are maintained over any length of time, as American studies found that substantial differences between trained and untrained physicians tended to narrow and almost disappear over time (Peterson et al 1956). There do not appear to have been any surveys examining patient reactions to doctors before and after training. Bowling and Cartwright (1982), in their study of the elderly widowed, compared the widowed people's reactions to general practitioners who had undergone various types of training and found that doctors without any training were the ones most often felt to be very sympathetic. But as they point out, this was the one significant difference that emerged when a number of criteria were examined.

Professional preferences Mechanic (1968) carried out a postal inquiry of a random sample of general practitioners dealing with their satisfactions and dissatisfactions, the organisation of their practices, attitudes toward various aspects of medical care, work load and views on issues of relevance to the organisation of general practice within the National Health Service. After two reminders, he obtained a response rate of 60% to his lengthy questionnaire. He then sent a much shorter questionnaire to those who had not replied and an additional 13% completed this. Out of 26 items he asked about, those most frequently regarded as problems (by 60% of the doctors) were: the amount of time they had for each patient, incentives for the time-consuming complex case, amount of remuneration received, method of remuneration and adequate time for leisure. The least problematical areas were perceived as access to diagnostic services and equipment, opportunities for professional contacts with colleagues and opportunities to work in cooperation with health authority workers. Mechanic found that satisfied doctors were more likely to have smaller practices than dissatisfied ones but that satisfaction was not related in any substantial way to age or whether the doctor worked with partners or single-handed.

Mechanic constructed an index of doctors' 'social-psychological orientation' on the basis of three questions. These related to the frequency with which doctors let a patient talk for half an hour or more to 'get things off his chest', initiated discussions about psychological factors or spent half an hour or more exploring a patient's social and emotional background. He found that this index was related to a variety of attitudes and reports of 'behaviour indicative of a social orientation to medicine. For example, doctors high on the social-psychological scale were more likely to report a considerable proportion of their time spent on providing psychological supportive care.' This is hardly surprising. Such an association seems more of a circular argument than an illuminating finding.

Career preferences of doctors have been extensively studied. Parkhouse and his colleagues surveyed doctors graduating in 1974 (Parkhouse and McLaughlin 1976) and in 1975 (Parkhouse and Palmer 1977). The response rate was 86% in the earlier study, but in the later one names were not obtained directly from medical schools but were derived from the GMC's fortnightly lists of provisionally registered doctors, and the response rate was lower, 81%. There was a large increase in the proportion of responders giving general practice combined with some other speciality as a first choice: from 1.4% in 1974 to 12.1% in 1975, but as the authors themselves point out: '. . . it is difficult to escape the conclusion that the unpremeditated use of "general practice with hospital sessions" as an example in the questionnaire may have prompted a flood of responses in this direction'. As they say, 'here is a lesson, doubtless well-known to others, in the wording of questionnaires and a warning for all on their interpretation'. Preferences are analysed by sex and by medical school. Women were more likely to opt for community medicine and paediatrics as their first choice and few of them chose surgery. Nottingham had the highest proportion opting for general practice on its own and for community medicine. The proportion choosing geriatrics was not shown, presumably because so few did so.

Particular professional groups One group that has been studied fairly extensively is **women doctors**. Jefferys and Elliott (1966) considered the obstacles to employing them on a full-time or part-time basis in the health services. Beaumont (1978) compared their results with a survey in three Thames regions in 1976 and found that 'the results suggest that the professional commitment made by women doctors has increased over the past 15 years'. This would have been more conclusive if she had covered a wider geographical area or if the earlier study could have been re-analysed by region and the comparisons restricted to the same area. Beaumont (1979) also reviewed the provisions for women doctors to train and practice in medicine after graduation. Both studies were done by postal questionnaires and obtained responses of 75%.

More unusual are two studies relating to **male midwives**, one monitoring a training scheme in London which accepted male pupils as a pilot experiment; the other monitoring independently a somewhat similar experiment in Scotland (Speak and Aitken-Swan 1982).

The London study aimed at investigating the competence and capability of the male midwives, the costs in opening the profession to men, as well as acceptability to mothers, their husbands and staff. I have concentrated mainly on the acceptability to mothers. At the two hospitals taking part in the study mothers were interviewed at the booking clinic by the sister, who used a structured questionnaire to ask about the acceptability of care from male midwives. Mothers were told that the hospitals trained men, as well as women, to practise as midwives, but that 'chaperoning would be available and all men would be sufficiently trained for the tasks they had to do' (page 26). Mothers were then asked if they objected to that arrangement: at one hospital 17% did so, at the other 30%. Women whose nationality was described as Indian, Pakistani or Cypriot (it is not stated how this information was obtained or defined) were more likely to ask for female midwives – but this does not account for the difference between the two hospitals. Mothers were seen again by study interviewers as soon as possible after admission and on the day before discharge. There was less difference between the two hospitals in the 'rejection rates' of male midwives at these stages. On admission these were 17% and 21% and on discharge 16% and 19%. Rejection rates were lower among those who had met male midwives prior to admission and among those receiving care from male midwives during admission – but it is not clear which is cause and which effect. Presumably those who had 'rejected' male midwives at the booking in clinic were unlikely to encounter them in hospital, although this cannot be the whole explanation for the observed differences. Further analyses would have been illuminating.

Using data from ratings made by nursing officers, sisters and staff midwives who had trained pupils included in the study it was concluded that: '. . . male pupils in London have proved to be no worse than their female cohorts with respect to competence in practical work and capability at theory' (page 91). This was on the basis of six male pupils who started training in one year and two in the following year. Four of the eight are now State Certified Midwives, one died, one was asked to leave because of lack of competence, a third found the strain too great and discontinued and the fourth broke his leg and was still in training (page 25). No conclusion was reached about chaperoning.

The Scottish study focused on the 'social acceptability of male student midwives to women during pregnancy, labour and the puerperium, and to their husbands/consorts; as well as to midwives, obstetric consultants and registrars, and general practitioners participating in the maternity services'. I have again concentrated on the survey of mothers, 500 of whom were interviewed. The questionnaire was designed to avoid suggesting that there was anything strange about male midwives and aimed at finding out 'which nursing functions, if any, the mother would accept from a male midwife and which she would not wish him to perform for her' (page 47). So the subject was approached indirectly: the mothers were asked if they knew which were the student midwives and which the trained staff when they did things for them, what items of nursing care had been done by students and then how they had found the students. The assumption was that if mothers had been tended by a male student and had views on them one way or the other, they would bring the matter up without being asked directly. In fact, of the 248 who had come into contact with the male students or had had nursing care from them, only 15% mentioned their sex spontaneously and they did so 'casually and without emphasis' (page 52). A final question addressed the problem of sex directly and asked: 'Does it make any difference to you if you have a male or female midwife?' Fifty-seven per cent of the mothers said the sex of their midwives made no difference to them and in reply to a prompt they said this was so whatever the nursing procedure to be done; 4% found the idea of a male midwife wholly unacceptable and 35% unacceptable for intimate nursing procedures; the rest were undecided. Half the mothers had come into contact with the male students or had had nursing care from them, but there is no analysis in the published report of the views of the two groups.* A total of 1,951 women attending the booking clinic were asked this question: 'In this hospital we train both men and women midwives so you may have a man or women to give you all kinds of nursing care, such as bedbaths, fixing the baby to the breast and so on. Does it make any difference to you which you have?' Almost three-quarters, 73%, said it made no difference to them. No analyses are presented with their views obtained at an interview after the birth and it is unclear how many of the women were included in both parts of the study.*

---

* Analyses on these points are made in the full report which is 'available for inspection at the DHSS Nursing Research Division'.

The report on the two studies concluded that male midwives have been shown to be generally acceptable to mothers. This was the basic question addressed and answered. I think the fascinating thing about these studies is the concentration on that question. Women having babies accept many things which are increasingly being questioned by a variety of groups and movements. But was there a seriously considered possibility that there would be any noteworthy rejection of male midwives of women in labour? And once the male midwives had been involved in labour and delivery was it likely that they would be rejected at a later stage? And why was the acceptability of male midwives felt to be an issue when that of male medical students and male doctors is taken for granted? If the question to which the surveys had been addressed had been their relative preference for male or female midwives then a different study design would have been needed comparing reactions of women either before or after the introduction of male midwives or hospitals with or without them. The adopted design was appropriate for the particular question posed: this was concerned with the acceptance of a particular professional group – not with the preferences of patients. I do not think it was appropriate in the London part of the study to reach even tentative conclusions about the likely competence and capability of male midwives on the basis either of such small numbers or on the first entrants to such a scheme.

Other organisational studies

Probably the most influential series of studies in relation to the organisation of the health services were carried out by the Brunel Health Services Organization Research Unit. A book, *Health Services: their nature and organization and the role of patients, doctors, nurses and the complementary professions* edited by Jacques (1978), 'presents some of the main findings arising from the [Unit's] works' (page vii) and describes their mode of work – that of social analysis. No surveys are reported and as Klein (1978) puts it 'the book is surprisingly short of evidence about the actual operation of the NHS given that their method of work is to concern themselves with the practical problems of the service and to derive their conceptual models from experience. In the outcome we get a lot of models but precious little information'. Some surveys or other objective data would have been illuminating.

Since 1974, National Opinion Polls have conducted a regular series of polls for BUPA, looking at attitudes to private medical treatment and insurance. These are based on quota samples 'designed to be representative of all adults in Great Britain'. Among a series of questions to full-time employees they asked: 'How interested would you be in having private medical insurance for yourself and your family as a job benefit, if your employer was to provide it?' Their results suggested that the proportion who were 'definitely interested' had risen from 27% in April 1978 to 44% in March 1980 (NOP 1980). It is interesting that even at the later date more than half those questioned were rejecting a proposal that was presented as a benefit.

Methodological issues

The main methodological problems associated with international comparative studies are: the difficulty of organising surveys that are comparable in practice, the immense amount of work and resources needed to organise them effectively and the relatively small pay-off from general studies in terms of useful data with either theoretical or practical implications. With the more specific studies problems were encountered in identifying comparable professional groups (Mechanic 1972), in carrying out widely enough based surveys to justify generalisation (Kayser-Jones) and in interpreting differences in subjective assessments (Shanas et al). Of the studies reviewed the one with the most far reaching policy conclusions, Titmuss's, relied least on survey data.

In the other fields there were problems relating to:

Obtaining a representative sample of doctors for the studies of time spent on various activities in general practice.

An inappropriate sample for a survey of prescribing in general practice.

Low response rates in some of the surveys of junior hospital doctors and general practitioners.

The lack of a pilot for the survey of medical students and their training in family planning.

A bias created by giving a specific example in a survey of career preferences.

The use of techniques that were essentially unrepeatable in one of the surveys of prescribing.

Lack of figures to support some of the conclusions in the study of the management of hypertension.

Inappropriate conclusions in the London study of male midwives.

Lack of survey or other objective data in the studies by the Brunel Health Services Organization Research Unit.

In conclusion

Is this another field, like acceptability, in which surveys are likely to have a conservative influence, supporting the existing organisation? The implications of international comparative studies are likely to be radical for at least one of the countries studied – the doubt is whether they are likely to result in action. Studies of variations in care are also likely to have radical implications and here it seems rather more probable that some action may result. Surveys from the viewpoint of professionals can ask both radical and conservative questions and produce either type of answer. They can also fail to ask a lot of pertinent but threatening questions. Indeed the lack of survey data relating to many aspects of organisation is the main conclusion of this chapter. In addition to the areas in which few studies appear to have been carried out – such as variations in clinical practice and variations in organisational factors in hospital – there are a number of fields in which a single survey, in a limited geographical area or based on a biased selection of practices, has not been followed up by other studies. An example of this is the observational study of time spent on different activities in general practice. And the study of differences between teaching and other hospitals has not been followed up more recently or on a wider range of hospitals. Another gap is in the evaluation of professional training which has been pursued only in a limited way, with little or no attempt to relate it to patients' experiences. As Ashley, Howlett and Morris said – nobody has the facts.

9 *Methodological issues*

Carrying out a survey seems on the surface a relatively straightforward exercise requiring commonsense, some organisational skills and possibly a bit of professional, statistical advice. I hope my descriptions of some of the surveys in the health field have shown that it is not so simple as it may appear and that there are many pitfalls at all the different stages of a survey: conception, design, execution, analysis and presentation.

In this penultimate chapter I discuss the various methodological issues and illustrate them mainly from studies that have been described earlier. I have tended to highlight the things that can go wrong.

Formulation of aims

This is fundamental and should be the starting point of any survey. Basically at this stage two questions need to be answered: 'What question(s) do I want to answer?' and 'How can a survey help to answer this (or these)?' Sometimes, particularly in the epidemiological field, the first is straightforward, for example 'Does some specific thing cause lung cancer?'; it is the second question that is more problematic since surveys can rarely answer such epidemiological questions unequivocally though they can, if carefully designed, be used to build up an almost water-tight case. But most surveys in the health services research field are directed to more than one question. Even when the basic question seems straightforward, for example, 'Do stroke patients do better in specialised stroke units than in ordinary medical units?', there are important supplementary questions: 'In what way?', 'Which patients?', 'At what cost?', which need to be formulated if the survey is to produce useful information.

It might be argued that descriptive studies do not aim to answer questions, but I think this is fallacious. Before such a study can be appropriately designed, the parameters of the description have to be decided, and this can most effectively be done by formulating questions. So in a descriptive study of a service these questions might be posed: 'How many people use it?', 'How does the proportion using it vary with age, sex, social class, attitudes, previous experience, and so on?', 'What conditions do people using the service have?' An alternative series of questions might be: 'What do the users see as the possible alternatives to the service?', 'How does this compare with the views of the professionals providing the service?', 'What do the users and the professionals see as the relative advantages and disadvantages of this service compared with the possible alternatives?'

An important part of the process of formulating aims is a search of the literature and of other studies in the field. Replication of research is often desirable, but it should be undertaken deliberately, not in ignorance. Indeed, effective replication demands careful analysis and understanding of the aims and methods of the study to be replicated. An ability to make comparisons with other studies can illuminate differences between areas and organisations and reveal trends over time. This last opportunity was disregarded in a study of patients' attitudes to hospital care (pages 99–103). Then findings of other studies should obviously be taken into account when formulating aims. I write 'obviously', but earlier study findings appeared to have been ignored in the series of surveys of drug prescribing by general practitioners (pages 123–125).

Clearly, the design of the study depends on its aims, and one common reason for inadequate or inappropriate design is failure to formulate the study's aims adequately. An example of this in the surveys I have discussed is the study of accident and emergency services (pages 64–66).

Study design

Nearly all the studies I have discussed fall into three broad groups in relation to their basic design: experimental studies on randomised controlled groups; prospective or follow-up studies which may involve comparisons but not of matched groups and finally, the largest group of all, retrospective studies which are descriptive but most of which also involve some comparisons.

The experimental studies based on randomised controlled trials might seem the most straightforward and least problematic of the designs. In practice there are many pitfalls related to exclusions, inadequate numbers, lack of blindness, treatment of controls and interpretation. Often it is only for certain groups that a trial is felt to be both appropriate and ethical. In the study of the management of stroke in the elderly (pages 71–76) it was not thought appropriate to include either those likely to do poorly, whether they were rehabilitated or not, or those likely to recover spontaneously. With the studies of tonsillectomy (page 77) it was felt to be ethical to include only children for whom the value of the operation was considered equivocal. Exclusions should be made on well defined criteria, and these criteria and the numbers of exclusions which result need to be clearly stated in the presentation of the results – which did not happen in the first reports on the study of the management of stroke in the elderly (pages 71–76). Ideally the effect should be evaluated by someone who does not know whether the person is in the treatment or control group, and the control group should receive an appropriate placebo. In practice this is not possible for treatments involving operations or admission to institutions. And in the study designed to affect the use of general practitioner services for specific symptoms (page 68) the interviewer did not know initially whether the person belonged to the treatment or control group, but this always emerged towards the end of the interview in response to certain questions and of course the respondent might mention it earlier. Further, the treatment given to the control group is crucial. There have been criticisms of the treatment given to the control group on the tonsillectomy trials (page 77). Ironically, the study that fulfilled all the appropriate criteria for the design – the clinical trial of clofibrate (pages 92–93) – ran into some of the biggest problems of interpretation because the authors took account of adherence to the drug regimen.

But probably the greatest difficulty in setting up randomised controlled trials has been objections on ethical grounds. However the view that it is *unethical* to embark on the widescale use of drugs or procedures *without* a proper trial is now more generally accepted. While current innovations are likely to be evaluated, there is the problem that it is still viewed as unethical to evaluate procedures that have become accepted without proper trials. But even in this field there is movement. I understand that the National Perinatal Epidemiology Unit is to carry out a trial of episiotomy.

The other point that needs more widespread acceptance is that surveys of patients' views should be part of the experimental trials. Measurements of morbidity or mortality are inadequate on their own. Assessments of treatment should also take account not only of physical side effects but of the social costs of attending for treatment, and the possible anxieties created. When there is a change of emphasis from institutional to community care, surveys of the relatives, friends and neighbours providing that care are needed to assess the implications of the changes for them. The appropriateness of the experimental design depends on measuring all the relevant effects. Experimental studies have been done on the use of services and on both the effects and acceptability of services. In theory it would also be possible to carry out an experimental study on some types of organisation, allocating some patients to care organised in one way and others to care organised in another.

Prospective and follow-up studies. These mainly involve defining the people to be studied and then setting up the organisation to interview them when they use the particular service or develop the particular condition, or when the appropriate interval has elapsed.

Examples of this approach are the studies of people becoming physically impaired (pages 63–64), attending accident and emergency departments (pages 64–66), having repeat abortions (pages 66–67), receiving medicines regularly (pages 90–92) using the ambulance service (pages 82–83) having a colostomy (pages 79–81), having a baby with Down's syndrome (page 82), becoming pregnant (pages 106–110), being in a hospital which trained male midwives (pages 135–138). Basically, these studies were descriptive – showing what sort of people were involved and/or their experience and views. Some comparisons were made within the groups, for instance of mothers with younger or older Down's syndrome children and of women who developed different types of postnatal depression. Problems arose over comparisons with groups that had not been studied. The authors of the study on accident and emergency services were tempted into making inappropriate comparisons. With repeat abortions comparisons were made with BPAS patients for marital status and occupation but no comparative data were available for contraceptive use and the problems associated with it. This would have been illuminating in view of the finding about the high incidence of side effects from oral contraceptives in the group studied.

Two prospective studies had a rather different design. The second study of lung cancer and smoking involved obtaining data about smoking habits from doctors and then following up by records to find out which ones had died (page 28). The other study also involved initial intervention and then observation. This was the study in which patients with inoperable cancer were told that after investigation they would be given truthful clearance or a firm diagnosis if they cared to ask (page 49). The aim was to find out what proportion asked; no attempt was made to identify characteristics related to asking or not asking.

As with the experimental studies, these follow-up surveys have been used to illuminate the use, effects and acceptability of services. In addition they are used to identify factors associated with disease and in organisational studies. They could also be used to follow up doctors receiving certain types of training or people cared for under different types of organisation. But of course such studies would be better done with an experimental design allocating the doctors or patients to the groups at random. If this is not practicable and ethical, there is the problem of ensuring that the two groups are comparable to start off with, or that any relevant differences between them can be controlled in the analysis.

Retrospective studies The majority of surveys discussed in this review fall into this category, and this type of survey is used in all the broad subject areas discussed. Although most of the studies on effects of care are either experimental or prospective, it is possible to identify groups that have been treated in the past in different ways and then ask about subsequent events. The main methodological problems associated particularly with retrospective studies are memory distortions and ensuring appropriate comparisons.

Much has been written and some data collected about **memory errors.** Slater (1946), Stocks (1949), Gray (1955), Douglas and Blomfield (1956), were some of the earlier writers with data on this; more recently Moss and Goldstein (1979) edited a book, *The recall method in social surveys.* Some of the practical points that have emerged are:

> When asking people about events over a defined period of time, a period ending on the day before interview is to be preferred as this prevents transfers in and out of that end of the period (Gray 1955).

> The more important the event to the respondent, the more likely it is to be recalled. Douglas and Blomfield (1956) found that mothers were least likely to forget illnesses that had occurred early in their child's life even though they were recalling these over a longer period.

> To reduce memory errors, information about some facts can be asked in two different ways and any inconsistencies identified and checked with the informant, for example, date of birth and age of children, gestation and date of last monthly period.

It would seem that the more important an event, the longer the period over which people can recall it with reasonable accuracy. So when a survey covers events of differing importance occurring with varying frequencies it is tempting, and may seem logical, to vary the periods over which people are asked to recall these different events. But this may be confusing. For example, the 1982 GHS in the section on health asks people first about their health over the *last twelve months*, then about restrictions in the *two weeks ending yesterday*, about any discussion with a doctor (apart from any visits to hospital) during the two weeks ending yesterday, about any casualty and out-patient departments during the months of _____, _____, and _____ (the *last three calendar months*) and about any in-patient stays in hospital during the *last year*. Those aged 65 and over are also asked about the use of certain listed services *last month*, and then about other listed services *last year*. I wonder about the effect of changing the recall period in this way.

There is also the problem of selective memory. The inquiry into the availability of doctors in emergencies (pages 96–97) asked about attempts to contact the doctor outside surgery hours in the last five years. I would expect a substantial bias in the response – the more dire emergencies and catastrophic outcomes being more readily recalled.

Turning to the problem of making appropriate **comparisons** in retrospective studies, five types of difficulty arose:

1 That of obtaining suitable controls. This occurred in the retrospective study of lung cancer patients (pages 24–26, 40), in which they were matched with other hospital patients, but this led to difficulties in making urban/rural comparisons. In the study which matched users and non-users of the general practitioner service by age, sex and the experience of a particular symptom, 82% of the interviews with potential controls could not be included (page 59).
2 Inability to make comparisons on the characteristics for which the controls have been matched. Controlling for age and sex was appropriate for the lung cancer and smoking study because it was not concerned with age and sex variations. But for the study of whether a general practitioner had been consulted about a particular symptom, age and sex may be the main explanatory variables; controlling for them precluded the exploration of this possibility in the study of matched users and non-users (page 59).
3 Studies covering only part of the population. International compa-

rative studies can only be used for international comparisons when they are based on national samples. Some of the studies did not attempt this, one had difficulty in achieving this (pages 117–119).

4 Obtaining appropriate indices of morbidity in order to interpret social class differences in use of services. This was apparent in the analyses of the GHS (pages 12–14).

5 Making comparisons between two groups of people without possibly biasing the study by identifying the characteristic by which they were to be compared. This was confronted in the studies of the menopause (pages 32–35).

Sampling

This is discussed under four headings: sampling frames, sample design, sampling procedures and sample size.

The sampling frames that are generally available for samples of people, households, addresses or dwellings are the electoral register and the valuation lists. Some of the problems related to the **electoral register** are that only people aged 18 and over, who are British subjects (that is, including Commonwealth citizens) or citizens of the Republic of Ireland and who are resident in the area on the qualifying date, are included. Some studies have suggested that between about 3% and 7% of eligible electors are not registered to vote and that omissions are most marked for persons who attain the minimum voting age during the currency of the Register, Commonwealth citizens, naturalised British subjects, boarders, tenants and people in institutions such as hospitals and old people's homes (Gray, Corlett and Frankland 1956, Gray and Gee 1967, Newton 1976).

A more recent study in five registration districts of London showed that of women who had recently had a baby in those areas only 61% were on the electoral register. Some will have been ineligible – omissions were most marked for young, single and working-class women (Smith 1981). So for data about inequalities relating to social class, race or country of origin the register of electors may be a less than satisfactory sampling frame for the selection of individuals, although there are ways of overcoming some of these disadvantages which will be discussed under sampling procedures. The GHS sample is drawn from the electoral register but the unit is addresses. However, addresses at which no individual is registered will not appear so those containing only people under 18 or non-British people will automatically be excluded. Others may be omitted because of inadequacies in the register.

Hereditaments, that is buildings or parts of buildings that are rated separately, are the units in **valuation lists**. They can be used as a basis for obtaining samples of households as long as an appropriate procedure is adopted. Valuation lists are available only for local authority districts whereas electoral registers are arranged by polling district, ward, local government district, parliamentary constituency and county.

A third possibility for a general sampling frame is the **postcode address file** which has only recently become available. Its advantages and limitations have been discussed by Leivesley, Breeze and Owen (unpublished). It has almost complete cover of addresses but includes a relatively large number of ineligible addresses.

Other national sampling frames are the register of deaths, used in a study of the needs of the dying (pages 47–48) and one of widowed people (page 134), and the register of births which was used in a study of childbearing (page 106). It is also possible to obtain national samples of marriages (Peel and Carr 1975). Access to a comprehensive list of divorces is obtainable only through the Lord Chancellor and I have not come across any studies related to health or health care based on this, but I understand that it has been used for at least one legal study (Murch 1980). Abortions are notified nationally but of course there is no available register.

Another method of obtaining a sample which claimed to be national was through a television programme. This identified a number of mothers who had recently had a baby (page 110). Such an approach can yield impressive numbers, but interpretation is difficult in numerical terms. Bias in relation to social class or marital status or mother's age could be established. It is also possible that women who were critical of the way they were treated in pregnancy or labour may have been particularly likely to respond to the invitation to take part in the study in the hope of exerting some influence. Nevertheless such studies can illustrate the sort of problems that arise – though estimates of frequency must be treated with extreme caution.

Most studies of needs are based on population samples since they are concerned with those who are not receiving care as well as those who are being cared for. General studies of health and sickness are also based on national population samples, as are some of the surveys on accessibility of care and satisfactions with care. And survey methods can be used to identify groups for more intensive study such as the disabled, the elderly, women of childbearing age or smokers.

For studies in general practice, age-sex registers can provide a useful sampling frame, as in the study of the prevalence and outcome of female sterilisation (pages 83–84). But by no means all practices keep such a register and they need to be kept up to date. There is also the problem of access to such records being restricted to the doctors who set them up.

A number of the surveys discussed in this review were based on samples of people receiving care. Hardly any surveys based on such sampling frames attempt to be nationally representative. One of the few that did was the survey of abortion patients carried out for the committee on the working of the Abortion Act (Cartwright and Lucas 1974). Usually, they are based on particular hospitals or practices. Even attempting area studies from such a basis presents considerable problems, in terms of, first, the sample design and, secondly, obtaining access to the information. The approval of ethical committees has to be obtained and often the consent of several different bodies is required. Since access is through the professionals providing the service there is an immediate likelihood of bias on issues related to the willingness of professionals to allow access to the information. In practice, quite a number of the surveys based on particular hospitals have been carried out by the professionals providing care. The ethical considerations of this and of giving other research workers access to samples of patients are discussed later.

For sampling doctors one possible source of information is the British Medical Register. This was used for the prospective study of lung cancer and smoking (page 28). But for studies concerned with practising doctors the register has many disadvantages since people who have retired or are not working for other reasons, and those in purely academic, research or teaching posts, will also be included. The only information it gives is the person's sex, qualifications (with date) and registered address. The Medical Directory contains some information about current jobs but has a less complete cover, being based on returns to an 'annual schedule' sent to those on the Medical Register. The response rate is not quoted.

The DHSS has information about doctors working in the NHS and could provide lists of general practitioners and of consultants in different specialities but it is difficult to maintain up-to-date lists of housemen and registrars because of their mobility. The willingness of

DHSS to supply lists will depend on their assessment of the researchers' credentials and agreements about confidentiality. Other possible sources of information are Family Practitioner Committees for general practitioners, regional health authorities for hospital doctors. When information is obtained through committees or individuals there are the problems of sampling these initially and then obtaining their cooperation. An alternative approach for identifying a sample of general practitioners is through patients. This was done in the survey of the needs of the dying (pages 47–48). When this method is used, the chance of a doctor being included is related to the number of patients who regard him or her as their doctor and on their willingness and ability to identify the doctor.

Medical students were identified by the Deans of Medical Schools in one instance (page 132) and by local representatives of the British Medical Students Association in another (pages 132–133). For the study of community nurses (pages 129–131) the 24 health districts which cooperated in the study provided complete lists of district nurses, community midwives, health visitors, school nurses, family planning nurses, 'joint duty staff', clinic nurses and community psychiatric, geriatric and liaison nurses. GP practice nurses were identified by 89% of the general practitioners in the study areas. The study was done by the Office of Population Censuses and Surveys and district nursing officers may be more willing to cooperate in that sort of way on such official studies than on studies carried out by less prestigious organisations. Persuading people to give access to the necessary information takes time and a lot of personal relationship work.

Sample designs Most of the national samples discussed have been two-stage or multi-stage: first of all, areas (or hospitals) are sampled and then individuals or households within them. The reason for doing this rather than straight random or systematic sampling throughout the population is that straight random sampling would lead to such diffuse samples that interviewing costs would be unacceptable – although this would not be a problem for postal studies. But with postal studies, if a check is to be made on the possible existence of either false positives or false negatives, or on non-responders by interview, then some clustering is needed.

The basic principle in designing a two-stage sample is that if equal numbers of people or households are to be approached in the selected study areas or hospitals, the areas or hospitals should be selected with probability proportional to the number of such units (people or households) that they contain. An alternative sampling strategy is to give each study area an equal chance of being included in the survey and then use the same sampling fraction for selecting people or households in all the study areas. In this way, larger numbers are selected from the larger areas and smaller numbers from the smaller. Either of these two methods gives a random sample with each final stage unit – people or households or whatever – having an equal chance of being included. This is achieved by the balancing of the two probabilities of the first and second stage units being included. If areas are chosen with probability proportional to population and then the same sampling fraction is used in all areas for selecting people, the result will be a biased sample with people from larger areas having a greater chance of being included. In contrast, if all areas have an equal chance of being chosen and similar numbers are selected within them, those in smaller areas have an unduly high chance of being chosen. The survey on short stay residential care of the elderly (pages 112–113) fell into this trap.

Multi-stage sampling designs lead to larger sampling errors than simple random sampling. But sampling errors can be reduced by stratification – listing the areas or hospitals by some relevant characteristic. This improves sample design by building in the appropriate representation and not leaving it to chance. For example, in the survey of family planning services in England and Wales (pages 61–62) registration divisions were grouped into those mainly served by 'good', 'bad' and 'other' services. This ensured that appropriate proportions of areas with these types of services were included in the study. Such directly relevant characteristics are often not available. For the GHS, which is currently based on a two-stage design and uses wards as the first stage units, wards are stratified first by region, then by metropolitan or non-metropolitan areas, thirdly by socio-economic group, and finally by the proportion of owner-occupiers. The GHS changed from a three-stage to a two-stage design in 1975. Some change had to be made then because of the reorganisation of local government but a two-stage design was adopted to reduce the effect of previous clustering. This had led to relatively high sampling errors in the variables relating to households and their accommodation.

An indicator of the design effect of a sample is the ratio of the sampling error for that design to the estimated random sampling error in a simple random design. For the GHS in 1976 this ranged from just under 1.0 to 2.09 for the variables for which it was calculated. In general, the design effect was smaller in 1976, with the new sample design, than in 1971, as expected. But apart from the GHS and the survey of the needs of the dying (pages 47–48), sampling errors in the national studies with complex designs are not published. I think they should be for at least some of the main study variables.

For one survey neither of the two basic designs for a two-stage sample was appropriate. This was a survey of abortion patients (Cartwright and Lucas 1974) and the problem was the wide variation in the number of abortions carried out in hospitals and clinics. To get a representative sample of abortion patients it was first necessary to sample hospitals and clinics in which abortions were performed. But over a third, 36%, of these institutions carried out less than ten in a quarter and altogether they did only 3% of all abortions. At the other end of the scale, 9% of the institutions did 100 or more and 64% of all abortions. To sample the institutions with probability proportional to the number of abortions they carried out and then take equal numbers of abortions from each of those chosen, would have meant waiting indefinitely for some of the institutions to accumulate an adequate number. Alternatively, to give all the institutions an equal chance of being included and then sample abortions in proportion to the number done (for instance by taking all the abortions within a particular period of time) would have meant almost all the survey abortions being taken from just two or three institutions. To overcome this difficulty, institutions carrying out abortions were divided into two groups, those doing less than 50 abortions in a quarter and those doing 50 or more. The first group was sampled with equal probability and then all the abortions occurring in a four week period were eligible for inclusion in the sample. The second group was sampled with probability proportional to the number of abortions they performed and then 20 patients were sampled from each of the institutions selected. The sample was designed so that the appropriate ratio was selected from each of the two groups.

Quota sampling was used in the NOP studies for BUPA (page 139). The advantages are speed and cost, but the disadvantage is uncertainty about the estimates since it it not possible to calculate sampling errors and there may be biases in the way informants are selected. Interviewers are normally told how many men and women to interview in three age groups (18–34/35–54/55+) and three social class groups; that is, the number in 18 groups are specified. The survey for

BUPA was done in 'over 200 sampling points throughout Great Britain' and in 1980 8,279 adults were 'interviewed at home'. NOP also do a 'random omnibus survey' every week except Christmas and Easter. It would be interesting to know how estimates from the quota samples compare with those from the random ones.

Sampling procedures The process of selecting areas with probability proportional to population is a simple one. The areas are listed in the appropriate stratified order together with their populations and these are summed cumulatively. If the total population is N and n areas are to be selected the sampling fraction is $^N/n$ and a number under this, x, is selected from a book of random numbers. The areas in which x, x+ $^N/n$, x+ $^{2N}/n$, and so on fall in the series of cumulative population totals then become the study areas. If the sample is of deaths or births or households or adults it is obviously preferable to select the areas with probability in proportion to deaths or births or whatever. The procedure is similar.

Sampling individuals from the register of electors is straightforward, care only being needed to exclude Service voters – marked with an S – and those who had not reached 18 on the qualifying date – marked with a Y. (It is inappropriate to include these because they are inadequately represented.) But there is the problem of people who are not registered as electors and of those who have recently moved. A technique for overcoming this has been developed by Blyth and Marchant (1973). This involves listing all the people at the selected addresses in addition to those on the electoral register. This listing has to be done in a specified order, for example by age, because selected individuals have to be interviewed. Problems can arise with starting an interview in this somewhat inquisitorial fashion. The theoretical advantages need to be set alongside the practical difficulties.

For sampling households the usual procedure, adopted by the GHS, is to use the electoral register to obtain a sample of addresses. All households at those addresses should then be included in the sample. In practice, interviewers are instructed to interview a maximum of three households at any one address and if there are more than three to select three 'by taking the first three surnames in alphabetical order.' To compensate for these additional interviews, other addresses on the interviewer's list are deleted – chosen by taking the one with the next largest serial number on which the interviewer has not already called. In theory these procedures could produce some biases, against households living more than three to an address, against people with surnames towards the end of the alphabet, and against people in addresses that interviewers left to the last to call on. In practice these biases are almost certainly negligible although it would be useful to see this demonstrated. But if every nth person on the register or every nth surname was chosen and then the households in which these fell were included, the sample would be biased towards households with most people or those with more than one surname (See Gray and Corlett 1950).

Samples of children are sometimes obtained (as on the GHS) by including all those in households; on other occasions samples of individual adults may be questioned about their children. In the latter instance there is the danger that children in single parent families may be under-represented while those without any parents may be left out altogether. This last happened with one of the studies of incontinence (pages 51–52) but is probably a small bias.

In obtaining samples of consultations or other events it is important to include all those taking place during a specified period of time: selecting the most recent is likely to result in bias (pages 94–95).

The procedure of a postal screen to identify samples of people with particular characteristics has been used in a number of the surveys described in this review. When two reminders are sent this usually gives a response rate of around 85% and is a useful technique.

Sample size Text books about surveys usually give the formula for calculating the sample size. This is based on an estimate of the variable to be studied and, in the case of a mean, its standard deviation. (See, for example Moser and Kalton 1971). The acceptable standard error of the estimate is also required. It is rare that researchers know so precisely what they are looking for and its likely variation. Among the surveys discussed in this review only those concerned with the prevalence of incontinence (pages 50–52) had as their main aim the estimation of the frequency of a single characteristic. If analyses by sex, age and parity are required then the sample size will be considerably larger and further assumptions and calculations must be made.

For a study such as the one on smoking and lung cancer, calculating the required size depends on estimating probable differences in death rates between smokers and nonsmokers. This is clearly important, otherwise real differences may exist but be statistically insignificant in the samples studied.

Surveys in the health field rarely make claims for differences that are not statistically significant at the 5% level. One exception mentioned in this review (page 82) and quoted in *The Times* as showing a difference between parents of younger and older children with Down's syndrome, was in fact based on such small numbers that the apparently large difference did not reach a level of statistical significance. A more common error is to conclude that there is no difference on the bases of samples which would only have detected very substantial differences. An illustration of this is the comparison of patients treated surgically or by injection/compression schlerotherapy for their varicose veins (page 113). Initially, 100 patients were treated surgically and 115 by injection/compression. At the three year follow-up, 90 of the former group and 110 of the latter were interviewed and it was concluded: 'The results at three years after treatment showed no difference between the two methods of treatment.' (Chant, Jones and Weddell 1972). This was on the basis of 14% of those in the surgical group and 22% in the injection/compression group needing further treatment. At the five year follow-up, 24% of those treated surgically had been given further treatment compared with 40% of those treated initially by injection/compression schlerotherapy, and the conclusion was that the probability of having no further treatment is greater for those treated surgically (Beresford et al 1978).

But adequate sample sizes, correct sampling procedures and appropriate sample designs are to no avail if the response rates are inadequate. These are discussed next.

Response rates

I discuss these under five headings: 1 response of general population to interview surveys; 2 response of general population and of patients to postal studies; 3 response of patients to research interviews; 4 response of health professionals to surveys; and 5 effects of non-response. But first there is the problem of definition. In some studies, response rates are presented in terms of the proportion of the initial sample who participated. In others various exclusions are made – such as patients who died or proved to be ineligible. The circumstances and the appropriateness of exclusions vary but it means that the response rates on the different studies are by no means always comparable. In some surveys, non-response is synonymous with refusal, in others there may be a variety of other reasons for failure to obtain information.

Response of general population to interview surveys In the surveys discussed, which were based on interviews with samples drawn from the electoral register, response rates were generally in the region of 82% to 91%. One reason for this comparatively high response rate is, I suggest, the subject matter: health is a topic that people are concerned about. The survey in which health was only one of a number of topics discussed is the General Household Survey. For this survey, response rates by individuals are not published, only response rates by households. Presumably this is because it is not known how many eligible individuals there are in some of the households. In 1978, complete household cooperation was obtained in 71.5% of households, no response in 15.3%, leaving 13.2% as partial responders. I would have expected complete response rates to be higher in the smaller households, so that individual response rates would be somewhat less than 75%. But data in the 1979 GHS report (page 156 of report) suggest that response rates were higher in the larger than in the smaller households, so individual response rates may be nearer 80%.

One problem is that response rates are likely to be lower among the sick and the elderly. Some studies take 'proxy' interviews to try to minimise this bias, but this creates other problems particularly over data about perceptions and attitudes.

Other factors beside the subject matter which are likely to affect response rates are the organisation carrying out the survey, the experience, confidence and persistence of interviewers, the number and pattern of call-backs demanded by the organisation and then, possibly, advance letters. Few experimental data are available, and some of the factors are often confounded. For instance the Government Social Survey has a good record on response rates, but whether this is because their studies are perceived as official or important, or whether it is the experience and training of the interviewers, it is impossible to say. Organisations that do not insist on several call-backs at different times are unlikely to obtain good response rates – witness the general practitioner study discussed on page 91 which accepted a 38% non-contact rate.

One small experimental study which attempted to evaluate the effect of an advance letter was carried out on a sample of mothers and fathers of young babies (Cartwright and Tucker 1969). Letters were sent to a random half, telling them about the study and asking them to cooperate if one of the interviewers called on them. The response rate among the mothers was 91% and this was not affected by the letter.

The response rate among the fathers was less good, 82%, and for them the letter apparently increased the response rate from 77% to 88%.

Some interviewers like an advance letter, but others feel that it gives an opportunity for people to rehearse reasons for not participating: they prefer to start from scratch and argue that when people are confronted by a person they are less likely to consider refusing than when they receive a letter. My view is that the confidence of interviewers is important in obtaining a good response rate so it may be appropriate from the viewpoint of response rates to send letters when the interviewer prefers it, but to let others approach people without one. I have no data to support this.

An experiment on the General Household Survey with advance letters (Finch 1981) provided 'no evidence that the letters had either a beneficial or a detrimental effect on response. There was also no sign that the letter was particularly helpful to inexperienced interviewers in gaining response.' The letters were popular with most of the interviewers.

One consistent finding is that response rates are lower in London. In 1978 the 'middle response rate for households' on the GHS was 73% in Greater London and ranged from 79% to 88% in the other regions, being 82% overall. Possible ways to try and compensate to some extent for this persistent bias might be to increase the initial sample size in London or to weight the sample that was obtained.

Response of general population and of patients to postal inquiries At one stage it was thought that postal surveys were synonymous with poor response rates, but it is now recognised that with two reminders response rates of around 85% can usually be obtained. The Government Social Survey has done two reviews of the available data: Scott (1961) and Austin, Lewis and Scammel (1977). These indicated that the sponsorship of an official or respected body increased response rates, government sponsorship producing better response rates than universities, and universities than commercial organisations. In relation to response bias Austin, Lewis and Scammel conclude that the only point that seems to have been firmly established is that responders have a higher level of education than non-responders. But a study which investigated the potential bias in a mail survey of 2,471 disabled people with an 84% response rate (Sheikh and Mattingly 1981) found no significant differences between respondents and non-respondents in terms of education or duration of disability, though there were other differences. Sheikh and Mattingly suggest that patients who have something to complain about or report were more likely to respond to inquiries than those who had recovered from their impairments.

Several of the studies in this review used postal surveys to identify minority groups for later interview, for example the studies of the disabled (pages 43–45), the incontinent (page 51), hospital in-patients (pages 99–103), all with response rates of 86% to 89%. This approach might usefully have been used in the study of old people (pages 120–121) and would have saved around 5,500 screening interviews in the British part of the study.

In my opinion, the use of postal surveys could be extended, particularly when following up groups of patients. We have seen that a study of people discharged from hospital got a response of 62% without any reminders (page 104) while the survey of patients using an ambulance to attend an out-patient physiotherapy centre achieved one of 86% (page 83) when patients who had already been interviewed were given a stamped addressed postcard to record the time at the end of their treatment, the arrival of the ambulance and their arrival at home. It was not stated whether they were sent any reminders. The studies on the menopausal symptom based on general practitioner records got responses ranging from 68% to 92%, (pages 32–33), the one on incontinence 89% (page 50), and the one on female sterilisation, 97% (page 84). It may be that some part of this variation was accounted for by differences in the accuracy and up-to-dateness of the general practitioner lists.

Response of patients to research interviews When patients were interviewed while they were in hospital, response rates were stated in only a minority of the studies. In Doll and Hill's 1952 study, 85% of the 3,208 were interviewed; the main reasons for not interviewing them were that patients had already been discharged from hospital, were too ill or had died. No patient refused to be interviewed, although one interview was 'abandoned because the patient's replies appeared wholly unreliable'. In the controlled trial of the management of stroke in the elderly it was stated that all 311 of the eligible patients agreed to participate in the study. The implications are discussed in the section on ethics.

In the studies in which patients were identified in hospital but interviewed at home, responses varied from 100% in the study of colostomy patients (pages 79–80) to around 80% in the survey about becoming a mother (pages 106–110). In case this suggests that response rates varied with the extent to which the surveys were seen as an extension of their hospital care, I should point out that response rates were 97% in the study of the meaning of disability (page 63) while 7% of those followed up in the study of deviation from prescribed drug treatment (page 92) refused to be interviewed.

For the interview surveys of patients identified from general practitioner lists, responses appeared to be linked to frequency of consultation. This statement is based on the study comparing recent attenders with those who had not seen their doctor for ten years or more (page 58) in which response rates varied from 70% to 90% – 'dead' records having been excluded. The low response, 62%, on the compliance study (page 91) seems surprising. Since no patients refused, it may have been because of inadequate, poorly planned calls, or inaccurate lists.

To sum up the findings on response so far. In surveys carried out in hospital it would seem that nearly all patients participate, or the researchers do not record the refusals. In interview surveys of the general population, response rates on health surveys are around 85% and the response to postal surveys is similar. Response rates of patients to interviews in their homes seems to show a wider variation but there is no clear evidence of a higher or lower response compared with general population samples.

Response of professionals The response rate of professionals shows a wider variation, from 15% on the study of junior hospital doctors (page 131) to 95% of community nurses (page 129). In a paper analysing responses of 19 samples of professionals to studies carried out by the Institute for Social Studies in Medical Care (Cartwright 1978), I showed that responses were lower among doctors than nurses, that postal surveys of doctors appeared to lead to marginally lower responses than interview studies, and that there had been a decline in response rates by general practitioners over time. And an experimental study (Cartwright and Ward 1968) showed that both the length of the questionnaire and the sponsoring organisation affected response rates of general practitioners: they were more likely to reply to a questionnaire sent from a local university than to one from an independent research institute in London. The response rates from the studies discussed in this review roughly support these hypotheses.

I am puzzled by the relatively low (69% for men, 60% for women) response rate by doctors to the study of lung cancer and smoking (page 28). I would have expected more doctors to respond to an inquiry of that nature. One possibility is that the usual two reminders were not sent – but that would be surprising.

Clearly the response rate of 15% was unacceptably low, but one of 88% from a comparable group of doctors was obtained in the most recent review. (Review Body on Doctors' and Dentists' Remuneration, Twelfth Report 1982; Appendix). This was obtained by having interviewers in the hospitals who explained the study to the doctors and then collected the forms after they had been completed.

Obviously doctors and nurses are busy people and the increase in surveys in recent years is likely to have added to demands on their time. But surveys contribute to their professional knowledge and in this review I have attempted to show the many different ways in which they do so. It would be nice to think that this review might encourage a higher response rate among professionals!

Implications of non-response These vary with the aims of the study, as well as with the response rate. When the aim is to identify a small proportion of the population with a particular characteristic there is the theoretical possibility that all the people who did not participate might have the characteristic. For instance, in the study related to incontinence (page 52), although the response rate was high, 95%, if all those who did not respond had significant urinary incontinence this would about double the estimate of its prevalence. And it is at least plausible that a high proportion of people with this problem might be so embarrassed by it that they would not want to identify themselves.

But biases may go in either direction. One of the studies on disability (page 45) suggested that the disabled were more likely than the non-disabled to respond to the initial request of the postal inquiry than to wait for a reminder, although the other study in this field (page 43) reported no such difference. Other response biases that have been identified and related to the subject matter of the study were concerned with foot problems and consultation rates. Those who reported foot problems at interview were more likely to be willing to have their feet examined (page 53), while those who had consulted their general practitioner fairly recently were more likely to respond to an interview study about their health and attitudes to doctors than those who had not done so (page 58). And the response rate from junior hospital doctors was apparently highest among the doctors working longer hours (page 131).

These biases fit in with the hypothesis that response rates are higher when people are interested in or concerned about the subject matter of the study. This would suggest a high rather than a low response among the incontinent to the study mentioned earlier. People who do not have a problem may not realise that the researchers want to know that.

Often the only check that can be made is to compare the sample distribution with that of the relevant population in relation to such basic characteristics as age, sex and social class. However the fact that the two distributions do not differ significantly does not necessarily mean that there is no bias among the non-responders, even those with the compared characteristics. Cartwright (1959b), in a study where the marital status of those who were not interviewed was known, showed no significant difference in relation to marital status between the sample achieved and the sample as drawn, when the latter was used as a basis for population estimates. However, there was a clear bias when all the data were used – the single being significantly less likely to participate. Thus, insignificant differences in comparison with the population are not a guarantee of lack of bias, even over the characteristics for which such comparisons can be made. Some researchers seem unjustifiably confident about lack of bias in their samples on the bases of such comparisons.

Techniques of interviewing

In addition to identifying and tracking down the appropriate people to be interviewed, persuading them to cooperate in the survey and conforming to the ethical standards discussed in the next chapter, the interviewer using a structured questionnaire has three other basic tasks:

1 To ask the questions in the form and order laid down. This demands a thorough knowledge of the questionnaire, the definitions to be applied and any other instructions.
2 To listen carefully to the responses, asking supplementary questions when needed in an unbiased and appropriate form.
3 To record the answers accurately, fully and legibly.

A discussion of techniques is in the Government Social Survey's

Handbook for interviewers (Atkinson 1971). Situations that the interviewer needs to be able to cope with in a consistent and appropriate way are interruptions and contributions from people other than informant, recognising and dealing with inadequate answers, distinguishing a pregnant pause from an embarrassed silence and dealing with implied and non-verbal information. Four other aspects of interviewing that seem to me to need more discussion and clarification are how to deal with inconsistencies, how to cope with relevant information that is given before a question is asked, feedback, and the relationship between the interviewer and the person being interviewed.

Inconsistencies of facts need to be identified at the time by the interviewer and sorted out tactfully. Possible ways to do this are 'Can I check . . .', 'I don't seem to have got this down right . . .'. But people may well be inconsistent over their opinions and should not be challenged or confronted about them. In such a situation the interviewer should use such non-directive probes as: 'In what way?', 'How do you mean?', 'Could you say a bit more about that?' These can lead to clarification and views that initially appeared to be inconsistent become understandable and sometimes logical.

Information given out of order This arises with structured interviews and creates two sorts of difficulty. One is that relations with the informant can be upset if information already given, or views already stated, are apparently ignored by the interviewer. The other is that informants may merely give additional information when asked about something they feel they have talked about already, and not repeat what may be the basic information. The problem cannot always be avoided by the interviewer controlling the situation so that the informant never does this; it is impractical. Information is often given incidentally. To give a simple illustration: the question 'How old is your baby?' may be answered by 'He will be one next Thursday.' It would be an insensitive interviewer who went on to ask the baby's sex. To cope with the problem, the interviewer needs to pay attention to everything the informant says and to develop techniques for checking any factual data given out of order and for getting the informant to repeat relevant attitudes. On occasions the interviewer may need to say something like: 'You told me something about this earlier but I did not get it all down – would you mind going over it again?' The problem may be minimised or exacerbated by the questionnaire design and particularly by the order of the questions.

Feedback The ways in which – and the circumstances in which – interviewers react to and comment on responses of informants have been studied more in the USA than in Britain. Marquis and Cannell (1971) showed that the presence or absence of interviewer verbal feedback had a significant effect on the amount of health information reported in a household interview about family health, and Cannell, Marquis and Laurent (1977) have illustrated how verbal reinforcement by the interviewer can encourage adequate responses. They point out, however, that it is important to develop ways in which interviewers can effectively use reinforcement without introducing bias.

Relationship with informant The controlled relationship described by Cannell and his colleagues in their discussion of feedback is very different from the involvement described by Oakley (1981) in her work on motherhood. This may be partly because much of Cannell's interviewing is done on the telephone, but Oakley's feminist approach clearly contributes to the difference. She argues that 'when a feminist interviews women: (1) use of prescribed interviewing practice is morally indefensible; (2) general and irreconcilable contradictions at the heart of the textbook paradigm are exposed; and (3) it becomes clear that, in most cases, the goal of finding out about people through interviewing is best achieved when the relationship of interviewer and interviewee is non-hierarchical and when the interviewer is prepared to invest his or her own personal identify in the relationship'. Few survey researchers would go so far as Oakley; most would argue that it is appropriate for interviewers to avoid answering informants' questions at least until the end of the interview. But the issues she raises are important and need to be thought through.

Questionnaire design

It is difficult to write in general terms about questionnaire design without appearing to state blinding glimpses of the obvious. To do so is unproductive since people do not believe that they might fall into the trap of asking biased, ambiguous or inappropriate questions in an inappropriate order; nor that their questionnaires might not be able to cope with the different contingencies likely to arise, provide clear instructions and adequate space in which to record answers, be concerned with subjects which are meaningful to informants, or make it possible to analyse the answers efficiently and meaningfully.

Nevertheless, I think it is possible to find examples of a number of these failings in the surveys discussed.

Over **bias** I have not come across any blatant examples of the: 'You don't drink do you?' type, but I would argue that it was a form of bias to exclude the back or backache from the check list in the Survey of Sickness (page 6); and to obtain details only about the most recent consultation in the study of the accessibility of general practitioner care (pages 94–95).

The most blatant illustration of an **ambiguous** question seems to me to be: 'Will your doctor make home visits – always, never or sometimes?' (page 111), but there is also the ambiguity attached to 'you' (pages 95–96).

An example of what I see as an **inappropriate** question is the one to hospital in-patients: 'Did you feel that you could ask the doctors to tell you what you wanted to know or not?' (page 102) since many patients obtain most of their information from people other than doctors and, in addition, they are often told about things without asking. I would also argue that it is inappropriate to ask patients to recall attempts to contact a doctor outside surgery hours over a five year period (page 95) and that to do so is likely to lead to **bias** in the response.

On the **order** in which questions are asked, it can be debated whether general questions should come before or after specific ones. The argument for asking the specific ones first is that they can stimulate people to think about the topic and then the general question can summarise their views. I think this is often an appropriate and helpful approach, but it is open to the objection that mentioning specific things may bias general attitudes. Sometimes it is helpful to get informants' general reaction to an issue before asking specific questions. For instance an early question in the 1978 GHS section on health is: 'Over the last 12 months would you say your health has been good, fairly good or not good?' It would be difficult to ask that question in precisely those words after a person had gone into details of major illnesses during that time. One problem of asking the general question first is illustrated in the study of hospital patients (Gregory 1978) which started with a general question: 'Can I start by asking you, from your own experience as an inpatient would you personally say that on the whole the hospital service for inpatients is: very good, good, has its faults or is poor?' It would seem as if this question was used to start patients thinking, or to 'break the ice' with an acceptable start. But there is a danger that for some patients this will open the flood gates and they might want to pour forth all the difficulties they had encountered or talk about the superb way they were looked after. The interviewer then either has to cut them short – so the net result may be the opposite of that intended – or cope with a situation when a great deal of information is given out of turn in a form which makes it difficult to use.

One problem with postal studies is that respondents are likely to read through the questionnaire before answering any of it. This can introduce a bias. A way of overcoming a specific possibility of a bias was adopted in one of the surveys on the menopausal syndrome (pages 32–33). The questions asking directly about the menopause were in a second questionnaire, only sent after the first one on symptoms had been returned.

Some of the other difficulties encountered over formulating appropriate questions in a reasonable order were:

1 Developing appropriate questions and check lists for obtaining information about the general level of health (pages 5–7, 10–11).
2 Possible bias or variation introduced in time trends by adding additional questions on related topics which may stimulate people to think about their health and so affect their responses (page 12).
3 Deciding whether disability should be related to capacity or to performance (page 45).
4 Defining incontinence (pages 51–52).
5 Diffidence over asking single people about use of contraception (pages 61–62).
6 Ethical and humanitarian limitations over asking people about knowledge of approaching death (pages 48–49) and attitudes to handicapped children (page 82).
7 Obtaining reliable data about whether people had taken medicines prescribed by a doctor (pages 90–91).
8 Questioning people about things they did not know about (page 94).
9 Questioning people about attitudes to things they had not experienced (page 106).
10 Developing appropriate questions about different levels of anxiety and depression (pages 107–108).

Reasonable solutions were found to a number of these problems, others remain unsolved, and a few appear insoluble.

Classification and definition

Coding seems to me to be the Cinderella of the survey techniques. Relatively little professional attention is paid to it. Yet survey data can only be as good as the weakest process in their collection. A survey based on a proper random sample, with a high response rate and appropriate questions asked in the appropriate way by competent interviewers will be ruined if the data are not recorded and classified accurately. One study in this review in which this seemed to happen was the survey of the availability of general practitioners (pages (96–97).

Much of the coding of structured questionnaires can be done by interviewers on the spot. To do this effectively demands adequate piloting, careful wording and appropriate layout of the questionnaire, as well as competent interviewers. One potential disadvantage of 'precoded' questions is that interviewers may not record qualifications and doubts which respondents might voice in addition to the pre-coded response. But a well-trained interviewer will take account of these nuances in making the classification and it may sometimes be easier to do this than to record details fully for subsequent coding in the office. The Government Social Survey did an experiment on interviewer coding of occupation and industry (Hayman 1979). Field observations showed that interviewers often forgot to write down additional information which would have helped them to code with greater accuracy (McCrossan 1979). So the fact that the disagreement between interviewers and their 'Primary Analysis Branch' ranged from 11% to 30% does not necessarily mean that the interviewers classified responses wrongly in the same proportion.

Information about occupation is used to classify people's social class in nearly all health surveys and it reveals many fascinating differences. The theoretical basis for the classification is weak: social class is intended to indicate the 'general standing within the community of the occupations concerned', but the standing is not assessed on clearly defined criteria or on the basis of empirical research. Its attractions are comparability with other studies and national statistics and the fact that it appears to reflect meaningful variations. As the Central Statistical Office (1975) put it: 'It has justified its existence as a variable which highlights important differences that are related to the social position of the individual.'

One of its problems is the classification of women. Common practice is to classify married women according to their husband's occupation, single women according to their own occupation. But the social class distribution of men's and women's occupations is very different, particularly in relation to Social Class III, non-manual. The proportion of men in this group in 1971 was 11.9%, that of single, widowed and divorced women, 41.2%. When married women were classified according to their husband's occupation the proportion in this group was 11.3%, but when the classification was based on their own occupation it was 35.4% (Central Statistical Office 1975).

Other difficulties in interpreting social class data relate to changes over time and to differences with the age of individuals and the association between them.

The GHS uses a modified version of the Registrar General's Socio-Economic Groups for its classification of social class – collapsing it from 15 groups to six for most tables, and imposing a ranking on an unranked classification of occupations. The relationship between the classifications is complex and described in the Central Statistical Office article previously quoted. But the GHS classification must have similar problems in relation to sex, age and changes over time. The socio-economic comparisons in the GHS are presented for men and women separately and standardised for age, or presented separately for different age groups; but, in effect, for married and single women, chalk has been added to cheese. There is no easy solution and many of the other studies discussed adopt the same practice, sometimes without a break-down by sex, and occasionally (for example, in the study of compliance with drug prescribing in general practice, by Wandless et al described on pages 90–92) there is no discussion of the definition used or any mention of whether married women who work have been classified on the basis of their own or their husbands' occupation.

While many researchers use the same classification of occupation and social class despite its limitations, workers in the field of disability have tended to develop their own indices with a consequent loss of comparability. Thus, Patrick and his colleagues (1981) used a broader definition than Harris (1971) although Patrick incorporated Harris's criteria in a way which made some comparisons possible. However, Bowling and Cartwright (1982) in their study of the elderly widowed, used a shorter index related to mobility and to the ability to carry out various personal tasks. This made it impossible for them to compare the elderly widowed in their study with the general elderly population. Similarly, the 'nursing dependency index' used by Garraway and his colleagues (1981) for monitoring the progress of stroke patients was developed specifically for that study. The advantages of an index related to the needs of a particular study have to be weighed against the disadvantages of not being able to make comparisons with other studies. In retrospect, I think Bowling and Cartwright (1982) and also Cartwright, Hockey and Anderson (1973) in their study of people's lives in the year before their death made the wrong decision.

In addition to social class and disability another variable which can take up a great deal of coding time is illness. On the Survey of Sickness (page 7) conditions reported by the people interviewed were classified by staff at the General Register Office experienced in coding death certificates. All conditions and symptoms mentioned were said to be treated as separate conditions (Registrar-General 1955, page 6). How far this happened in practice may be questioned. Interviewers are likely to do the practical and apparently reasonable thing rather than to obey instructions implicitly – especially if they regard these as being theoretical and divorced from reality, and if they also involve extra work. The temptation to regard running noses, catarrh and coughs as all part of a cold and not to record them as separate complaints must have been great, and in many ways eminently reasonable. A method of linking associated symptoms seems desirable, and then there needs to be a way of identifying the main diagnosis.

In the first years of GHS from 1971–76 informants were asked: 'What do you suffer from?' if they reported any chronic condition; 'What was the matter with you?' if they reported that they had had to cut down on things they usually did because of illness or injury in the previous two weeks; and 'Why did you consult him?' for any consultations with the doctor last week or the week before. Diseases were coded according to the International Classification of Diseases using four digits 'under the supervision of the Medical Statistics division of OPCS'. There were additional coding notes for a number of terms not in the index. Results were published in 24 condition groups related to chapter headings of the ICD index but with a number of sub-sections. There was provision for up to four diseases to be coded at each of the three questions but no questions were asked at the interview to find which conditions the respondent thought were related, although the coding notes state that 'where a condition can be identified any symptoms of that same condition are ignored'. It is unclear how these were identified. Publication of the classification of diseases ceased in 1973 and in 1977 the questions were changed and check lists of conditions and symptoms introduced. The time, costs and difficulties of coding responses to open questions about illnesses almost certainly contributed to the decision to change.

Precoded questions certainly save time at the processing stage of a survey but they have other advantages too. They indicate to an interviewer the detail needed and therefore the amount of probing that is necessary. It is obviously unnecessary to find out whether someone was woken up in hospital before or shortly after 5 o'clock if the answers are both classified 'before 5.30', but if the initial response to a question is 'a doctor', a precode can indicate the need to distinguish between hospital doctors and general practitioners by probing. A neat way to overcome people's tendency to give answers to the nearest 15 minutes or so was used in Gregory's study of hospital in-patients (pages 99–103). The question 'how long did it take you to get to the hospital?' was precoded: '. . . about 15 (1–22) min/About 30 (23–37) min/About 45 (38–50) min/About 1 hr or longer (51 mins or more).'

Questions in which the possible codes are read out to the informant indicate not only the amount of detail needed but the possible dimensions of the reply. Another example from the study of hospital in-patients (pages 99–103). The question 'how long did it take you to have to wait . . .' was followed by prompted precodes: 'Longer than you expected/were you admitted sooner than you expected/or were you admitted more or less on time?' It might otherwise have evoked a response in terms of length of time. To construct appropriate pre-codes demands a full understanding of the possibilities and, particularly for questions of opinion, careful and fairly extensive preliminary or pilot studies.

My view about questionnaires that are made up entirely of precoded answers is that they are unsatisfactory for the respondent, the interviewer and the researcher. For the respondents it can be frustrating to be totally constrained in the choice of answer and to be unable to express things in their own terms. The relationship between the interviewer and the respondent is likely to be stereotyped and it puts the interviewer in an authoritative role that can be alienating for both sides. The researcher will be unaware of the different types of situations or opinions that are classified together and will not know about the difficulties and possible distortions involved in compressing them. Even if time and money constraints make it difficult or impossible to analyse any open questions I think it is helpful to include at least some. Not only can they be helpful in establishing good interviewer-respondent relationships but, appropriately worded and placed, they can improve the quality of precoded answers by giving the informant an opportunity to think more deeply about the subject. They can also provide at least illustrative material about what is included in the statistical data.

Analysis

If precoded questionnaires can lead to over simplification of the data, elaborate analyses can distance the researcher from the initial responses still further. Scales can summarise a series of questions usefully on occasions but sometimes one good question will do almost as well and then results can be presented more directly. I am particularly suspicious of factor analyses in which responses to a series of questions are combined in an elaborate exercise with dubious statistical validity and then given pretentious labels. Such techniques may be particularly tempting to researchers dealing with responses to questions of little interest and concern to the people being interviewed. Some pattern of response can usually be detected and, while it can be claimed that such techniques are more sensitive, I would argue that it is generally more sensible to adopt a more robust technique and stay closer to the data.

Few of the surveys discussed in this review adopted elaborate techniques. In the health field simple analyses are generally adequate although for some epidemiological studies, particularly clinical trials of potentially life saving or life destroying interventions, it is important to use sensitive tests and minimise the use of what emerge as inappropriate regimens.

But for most of the studies discussed in this review, straightforward analyses and simple tests of significance have been used. In theory, simple tests are not applicable to multi-stage sample designs and, as I have suggested earlier, I think more precise estimates of sampling errors should be made of key variables. Occasionally, further standardisation would also have been illuminating, for example the 1977 GHS analyses of illness and socio-economic group (page 19).

Both studies of the needs of the handicapped and disabled (pages 43–46) used responses to a series of questions to classify the disabled but did this in a clearly defined and straightforward way. Oakley (page 108) constructed a vulnerability index, but again that was simply done and contributed usefully to the interpretation. Mechanic's index of general practitioners' social-psychologic orientation (page 134) seemed less useful and indeed its associations seemed circular rather than helpful.

There are other problems in the interpretation of simple statistical tests applied to straightforward analyses. These arise particularly in the descriptive studies and stem from two aspects of the analyses: first, the stage at which hypotheses are formulated and, second, the number of analyses that are carried out.

In theory, hypotheses should be clearly formulated at the start of a study and in such surveys as the lung cancer and smoking survey (pages 24–31), the evaluation of stroke units (pages 71–76) and the study of clofibrate (pages 92–93) all of which relate to a basic single hypothesis, the hypotheses were stated and formed the basis for the study design. But in the more descriptive studies of the needs of the disabled and the dying, the surveys of dentistry and of family planning, those related to satisfaction and accessibility, and those concerned with geographical variations and professional views and practices, there were many ideas about the differences that might be revealed. In one sense there is a hypothesis behind each analysis, but these are seldom stated specifically – although I suspect the number of computer printouts might be considerably reduced if this were done. One danger of this approach is that it encourages significance hunting. Because the hypothesis has not been precisely formulated when the analysis is first examined, it seems, and indeed it often is, quite reasonable to group the data on the basis of the differences observed. Statistical tests are then applied and a level of significance attained. But strictly the tests are not applicable in that situation. I am not suggesting that they should not be carried out but that they should be interpreted circumspectly. They are a useful guide to likelihood of a difference existing or not, but in that situation they are not precise. The other implication is that before differences identified in such a situation are accepted they need to be explored in other studies.

Turning to the other problem of the number of analyses that are carried out, again this applies mainly to the descriptive studies, which often cover a wide range of variables, so that the possibility of many different associations can be examined. For example on the study of the needs of the dying (pages 47–48) over 450 items of basic information were collected. This means that over 100,000 two way analyses were possible. In fact only about 1,750 were carried out and a small fraction presented. Positive results are more likely to be presented than negative ones and in that situation it is theoretically possible for many of the differences identified as statistically significant to be ones that have arisen by chance. Researchers need to be aware of this possibility and to draw the attention of their readers to it. Again the main safeguard, too rarely used, is replication.

Validation

The survey researchers' nightmare is that interviewers might not bother to interview the right person or, worse still, they might complete a questionnaire without interviewing anybody. It is possible to arrange a call-back check on a proportion of the sample to check, first, that they were interviewed and then that they gave the same answers on the two occasions. That this happens in a proportion of instances may be a useful deterrent. A pleasanter solution, but one less easy to demonstrate, is to establish a trust between interviewers and the research organisation and build up a sense of job identification. I would hypothesise that payment on a salary or time basis, rather than by completed interview, helps to foster such a relationship. Inevitably, for random samples, a great deal of an interviewer's time is spent in tracking down the person to be interviewed and finding a convenient time for the interview. If, after spending a lot of time, the person refuses, or turns out to be ineligible, the interviewer may well have a sense of grievance about not being paid and may be tempted to interview someone else or even to make up the responses. If the survey is based on a sample of people selected from records, all the available and relevant information need not be given to interviewers. For instance when a sample of mothers is taken from the register of births the precise date of the birth and the baby's name need not be given to the interviewer but questions about these items can be included in the questionnaire. Any discrepancy can then be investigated.

This method, comparing data from interviews and from records, can also be used to check the accuracy of the data. But it cannot be assumed that the records are always right. Discrepancies may arise because of inaccuracies in the records, different interpretations, inadequate or imprecise definitions, and changes over time. In the survey of the needs of the dying (pages 47–48), three items of information recorded on the death certificate were asked about at the interview and coded independently – cause of death, age at time of death and place of death. Most discrepancies between the death certificate and the interview over the cause of death appeared to arise because the informant did not always have the information, or because the two sources differed in the selection of the main cause or the relatives more often gave old age or senility as a cause than the doctor who completed the death certificate. (At that time, old age was not acceptable to the Registrar General as a cause of death on the death certificate. I understand this has now changed.) Over age group at time of death, the interview data and the information from the death certificate tallied in 94% of instances, were one group out in 6% with no indication of a bias in one direction, and in three instances, 0.4%, there was a more serious discrepancy. These seemed to arise through ignorance. For instance a widow who gave the information on which the death certificate was based said her husband had told her he would be 45 next birthday, so the age at death was 44 according to the death certificate. But the Social Security people had subsequently told her that he had been born in 1913, so at the interview she placed him in the 55–64 age band. Discrepancies over place of death arose mainly from uncertainty about whether people died before they reached the hospital.

Another safeguard is to compare the distribution of answers obtained by different interviewers and check back on any who appear to be out of line. This can be helpful in identifying some misunderstandings or gross cheating, but is a relatively blunt instrument.

An ingenious use of other records to check survey data, but not information from individual interviewers, was made by Stocks for the Survey of Sickness (page 7). On the GHS, comparisons of consultation rates were made with data from the second national study of morbidity statistics from general practice (Royal College of General Practitioners 1974). The GHS rates are considerably higher than those in the National Morbidity Survey, particularly for the elderly. The possible reason for this, discussed in the GHS 1972 report, is the non-representative nature of the National Morbidity Survey. Other comparisons with GHS data were made with the 1971 census. These indicated that individuals living in Greater London were somewhat under represented in the GHS. Some of the other differences in relation to household size, age and marital status were thought to arise because of different definitions of household and the inclusion in the census of people living in institutions (OPCS 1973).

Another way of validating information is to interview people again at another time and ask them the same question. This technique was used by Doll and Hill to assess the reliability of smoking histories (page 25). The accuracy of the information and its stability are confounded in such checks. When such 'repeats' are carried out it is preferable for them to be done by different interviewers.

In a number of studies, the reliability of survey data was assessed by comparisons with information collected in other ways but specifically for the study. This technique was often used in assessing information about needs. On disability, responses to questions were compared with performance of tests (pages 43–44), and the impaired person's statement about the nature of the underlying medical condition was checked against the general practitioner's assessment based on notes and recollections (Warren 1976–see page 45). In one of the studies of incontinence a sample of those reporting it were interviewed by one of the survey nurses (page 51), while on the studies of feet and teeth problems (pages 53–54 and 59) people's assessments were compared with those of professionals. Surveys of compliance also frequently compared survey data with information derived from counting left over pills and, occasionally, with that from markers or stool analyses (pages 90–91).

Observation may be used to validate survey data; it can also be used to supplement it and give a different dimension. But most of the studies that have done this have been in the psychiatric field and therefore outside my sphere of interest. For instance, Clarke (1978) studied the care of patients on a long stay psychiatric ward for the elderly. She collected observational material of patients and interviewed nurses working in the same wards.

For the most part, concern to validate the information obtained in health survey data has concentrated around the medical data in the surveys. There are relatively few instances of re-interviewing people to check on the repeatability of their responses, or of employing such devices as asking the same question at the beginning and end of an interview. Another issue that has received scant attention in recent interview surveys in the health field is interviewer variability, and there are few reported assessments of the effect of presenting questions or check lists in different orders. These are problems that have been studied fairly extensively in the past and it may not be useful to collect further data about them now. Nevertheless, they need to be borne in mind when using survey data.

The final method of validation is by a further study to confirm the findings of an earlier one. This is rarely done by precise replication but in a number of the fields discussed here there has been more than one study and these second studies have, for the most part, confirmed and consolidated earlier results. This happened with the studies of the menopausal syndrome, the handicapped and disabled, the incontinent, the use of dental services, compliance with drugs and accessibility of general practitioner services. I have already indicated that in my view there were two fields (satisfaction with hospital services and variations in general practitioner prescribing) in which later studies did not build appropriately on earlier ones. In addition, there are a number of fields which do not appear to have had a second study to confirm earlier findings: the needs of the dying, trouble with feet, the health of non-users of general practitioner services, repeat abortions, evaluation of stroke units, follow-up of parents with Down's syndrome children, effects of ambulance travel, vulnerability to post natal depression, attitudes of blood donors, general practitioner management of hypertension, time study of consultations in general practice. All these studies seem to me to have yielded useful and important results which need verification.

Costs

The cost of a survey is related to many of the methodological issues that have been discussed:

The study design – the inclusion of control or other comparative groups – the distribution over time.

The sample – use of existing sampling frames – national or local samples – geographical clustering – size.

Response rates – the extent to which initial non-responders are followed up and other information sought in order to identify possible bias.

Techniques of data collection – postal or interview – open or pre-classified questions – simultaneous recording or tape recording and subsequent transcription – amount and complexity of data obtained.

Classification of data – amount of detail – construction of indices – independent classification.

Analysis of data – by hand, by 'counter-sorter', by mini or main frame computer – use of standard survey programmes.

Validation – checks on sample selection, on interviewers, on the consistency, reliability and repeatability of the data collected – independent checks on classification.

But it is hard to obtain reliable data about the costs of surveys and few studies have been done of the relative costs of different approaches. One of the problems is the extent and variation in hidden costs. Although a number of surveys are done under grants for specific amounts the additional costs are likely to vary enormously, particularly in relation to:

Overhead costs of accommodation and back up services (such as telephone, duplicating, postage, library services, typing).

Salaries of senior investigators, which may be covered by the university or other organisation in which the study is carried out.

Computing and other processing services.

Without detailed information on these points it is impossible to make useful comparisons of the initial estimated costs of surveys. And data about the actual costs with supplementary grants, extensions and other revisions are unobtainable for the majority of surveys. I think this is a weakness and researchers should give information about the costs of their studies. Funding bodies should demand them and publishers request them. In order to obtain comparable data, guidelines about the inclusion and ways of costing the items listed above would need to be carefully worked out and agreed. Although costs of health service research are small in relation to the costs of the services themselves it can be expensive to carry out careful surveys on representative samples, building in checks and validating the results. Scientific precision usually costs time and money. But knowing how much things cost in terms of money and resources is not only a useful tool of management but helps to put the value of individual surveys in proper perspective.

In conclusion

In this discussion of the methodological problems of carrying out surveys in the health field I have emphasised the things that can go wrong. If this bias is not recognised, this review could give a misleading impression. But in general the validation studies that have been carried out are reassuring and survey data often compare favourably with information from records or from routine statistics.

What can be done to minimise, or eliminate, inappropriate methods? The solution does not lie solely with the researchers, but also with funding, teaching and publishing institutions. A recent study investigated the reporting standards of 67 therapeutic trials published in four leading general medical journals – two British and two American (DerSimonian, Charette, McPeck and Mosteller 1982). This looked at eleven 'basic methodologic aspects that readers need to appraise the strengths of reported clinical trials', and found that out of the 737 items considered '56% were clearly reported, 10% were ambiguously mentioned and 34% were not reported at all'. These rates varied significantly between the journals: the *New England Journal of Medicine* reported 71% clearly, the *Journal of the American Medical Association* 63%, the *British Medical Journal* 52% and the *Lancet* 46%. The authors pointed out that editors have the power to control what is published and recommended that editors improve the reporting of clinical trials by giving potential authors a list of the important items to be reported.

This type of audit seems a useful exercise, not only for editors but for organisations that fund surveys and for the institutions under whose auspices surveys are carried out.

10 *The ethics, use and potential of surveys*

Ethics

Six stages of a survey seem to me to involve ethical considerations: deciding to do the survey, sampling, the collection of the data, contents of the questionnaire, data processing and the presentation of the results.

In **deciding whether to do a survey**, the researcher needs to have identified the questions the survey is intended to answer and how it is planned to do this. In addition, researchers should be sensitive to the possibility that they might be asked to do a survey in order to reduce pressure for action or to postpone uncomfortable decisions. Whether or not they decide to do the survey in such circumstances seems to be a decision with both ethical and political overtones. (The distinction I am making between ethical and political decisions here is that ethical ones relate to what is right or wrong, political ones depend on expediency and take into account what is likely to happen.) Determining whether or not a survey can answer the questions it is intended to is largely a technical issue: but deciding to undertake a survey when it cannot do so seems to me to be unethical if the researcher realises this, incompetent if he or she does not.

The issue of whether a subject should be researched seems to me political rather than ethical. When we decide we are, or are not, prepared to do research on ethnic, class, religious or sex differences, on variations between the public or private sector in health care, or, indeed, on any topic at all, we are making political decisions. And when we are anxious about the use which may be made of survey results I think these are political anxieties even though they may be about the unethical use of results.

Over **sampling**, there are no ethical problems about the use of public records such as electoral registers or rating lists. Use of the non-confidential part of birth and death certificates also seems to be relatively straightforward, although access to an appropriate sample of such records is dependent on the cooperation of the Office of Population Censuses and Surveys. If, however, a research worker wishes to select a sample from the register of births or deaths which is dependent on information from the confidential part of the record, there are practical difficulties and ethical problems. For example, the Institute for Social Studies in Medical Care recently wished to interview a sample of teenage mothers, but the age of the mother is on the confidential part of the birth certificate. It was suggested that the Office of Population Censuses and Surveys might select a sample which would include some unidentified older mothers. The interviewer would not know the ages of the mothers and therefore whether they were eligible for inclusion in the study or not. ISSMC felt that this met the requirement for confidentiality from the viewpoint of the individual mothers but it was decided at OPCS that this would be both unethical and illegal. Their solution was for their interviewers, from the Government Social Survey, to interview the sample, which still included a proportion of unidentified older mothers. This met their legal obligations but I think both the logic and ethics are debatable. By adopting this position, OPCS have given themselves a monopoly of surveys based on such samples. Perhaps the issue should be referred to the Monopolies Commission!

The census is another sampling frame of which OPCS has a monopoly. It was used for a study of people with nursing qualifications who were not at the time of the census employed as nurses by the NHS (Sadler and Whitworth 1975). As Alderson and Dowie (1979) put it: 'The adoption of this method of selecting a sample population created a considerable furore with questions about breach of confidentiality being raised in Parliament' (page 123 of their book). After this furore it was agreed that the use of any subsequent census for surveys, apart from studies to evaluate its accuracy, would be announced in Parliament, preferably before the census was carried out. I wonder about the ethics of that solution, but in practice it makes the use of the census as a sampling frame even by OPCS relatively unlikely. In any event, to revert to methodological rather than ethical issues, the census soon becomes out of date and other sampling frames from other studies are available to OPCS.

With samples selected from medical records, it is effectively the medical profession that has a monopoly. Doctors have been concerned with the ethics of experimental treatments and have built in careful checks administered by ethical committees. In many ways these seem over-elaborate when it comes to selecting and approaching samples for surveys since patients can refuse to participate simply by not answering questions. However, there is a danger that patients may think their care or treatment could be affected by non-participation. Safeguards are needed to ensure that this does not happen and that patients realise cooperation on surveys is voluntary and no penalties are associated with refusal to participate. In practice there are likely to be fewer misunderstandings when the research is conducted by non-medical rather than medical people, or when it is done by medical people not involved in care rather than by those who are. But it is those who are involved in care who can most easily obtain access to patients, and the non-medical researcher who finds it most difficult. Problems can arise in identifying patients with particular conditions or receiving particular forms of treatment, and it can be argued that it is unethical for names and addresses of such patients to be given to research organisations without the assent of the patients. What seems less clear is the nature of the assent that should be obtained. Should positive agreement be obtained or is it enough to notify patients that their names, and usually addresses, will be handed over unless they object? Certainly the latter procedure leads to higher response rates and in my opinion is reasonable unless the sample is based on data that patients are likely to feel is highly confidential, for example the fact that they had had an abortion or had a sexually transmitted disease. The problem is that what people see as highly confidential varies from person to person and over time. So in my view this is something of a problematic area. As with most ethical issues it is inappropriate to be dogmatic about this; there are conflicts of interests, for example, between scientific rigour and patient confidentiality, and where the most appropriate balance lies will vary in different situations. A guiding principle, as a recent *Lancet* editorial put it (1983), is that doctors should 'never divulge data revealed in confidence against patients' own interests'.

When follow-up interviews are carried out, or sub-samples of people from one survey are asked to participate in another, then it would seem appropriate to treat survey data with the same confidential constraints as medical records, so that the organisation who carried out the initial survey should do the subsequent interviewing too or they should get the agreement of participants in one study to their names and addresses being handed over to another organisation for a further inquiry. This is the stance adopted by OPCS who have used samples from the GHS and from their labour-force surveys for other studies.

Sometimes researchers obtain a sample from one source but feel they should seek the consent of a professional, usually the general practitioner, before approaching the individuals. It was suggested by some of the general practitioners approached that this should have been done on the study of the needs of the dying. Apart from the fact that this was impractical (since interviewers had first to identify the person who could tell them most about the last year of the person's life and had no idea who this might be, let alone who that person's doctor was), I think the suggestion is *un*ethical. People should be able to make up their own minds whether or not to take part in a study. To suggest that a doctor should veto who is approached is paternalistic.

Turning now to the **collection of the data** – either by interview or by post. Most, probably all, research organisations have a code of behaviour for their interviewers. At the Institute for Social Studies in Medical Care for example this says that interviewers should explain *who* they are, that is what organisation they come from, *why* the study is being done, *how* the person was chosen and *what* will be done with the information obtained. These points have to be explained by the interviewer before the start of the interview and in addition a written explanation is left with the informant. The amount of detail informants want will vary but it seems to me unethical to start an interview before making sure that there is no basic misunderstanding on any of these points.

It is important for informants to know what organisation the interviewer is from because otherwise they might answer questions under the impression that the interviewer was a member of the hospital staff, or from the Social Security or the local housing department or whatever. It is clearly unethical to obtain information under false pretences. I think it is also unethical to do so under false impressions of that nature.

In relation to the reason for the study, one important distinction to be made when seeking information from patients is whether it is wanted for research or needed for treatment or care. Inevitably there are overlaps and grey areas. Information about smoking may be helpful in making diagnoses and it may be wanted for research, but the person collecting it will almost always be doing so mainly for one reason rather than the other. Over treatment given in a clinical trial it may well be hoped and intended that the treatment will benefit the individual patient – but since they may be given a placebo and, in any event, there is some doubt about the beneficial effects of treatment, this needs to be explained. If a study is being done about a specific health problem or type of care I do not think it is unreasonable to present it in more general terms if the researcher wants to put the problem in a wider perspective.

In surveys conducted by post or in the patient's home I think people should, in general, be told where the interviewer got their name and/or their address. If it was obtained from medical records, the patients' permission should normally have been asked.

In most surveys, participants are assured that the information they give the interviewer will be treated confidentially. But this needs to be explained. ISSMC assures people that the information will be used for research purposes only and not passed on to anyone else and that in any report neither the people who take part nor the people they talk about will be mentioned by name, nor will it be possible to identify them.

In addition to giving people adequate information about the survey (who? why? how? what?) there are three other ethical aspects of interviewing. These relate to persuading people to participate, preserving confidentiality and responding to informants' needs.

Participation on surveys is voluntary and participants should realise this. At the same time a high response rate is important if the survey is to be worthwhile. So there is something of a conflict for interviewers and a potential danger that they might over-persuade people to take part when they do not want to. In practice I think that reluctant responders are rare, particularly on health surveys, and that interviewers soon acquire skills in persuading people to answer questions willingly. An initial hesitation is often overcome by explaining that people obviously need not answer a particular question if they do not want to. Problems can arise over the participation of patients in surveys carried out in hospitals or clinics or surgeries. It is less easy for patients to feel they have a right to refuse to participate in those situations than when they are visited in their own homes. The problem is accentuated if the interviewer has a professional relationship with the potential informant, such as that of doctor or nurse. I think such dual roles should be avoided if possible. And in my view such professionals should take particular care to make sure that patients realise they can refuse to take part. The lack of refusals in some of the surveys of hospital patients is, in my view, a cause for concern.

As well as not passing on any information about individuals, preserving confidentiality means treating questionnaires as confidential documents and making sure that no one outside the research organisation has access to them. All ISSMC interviewers and all ISSMC staff sign an agreement about observing confidentiality. Difficulties over confidentiality can arise when two people are interviewed and asked about the same situation – for example when patients and their doctors are interviewed separately but are both asked about the patients' conditions and circumstances. In such a situation it seems preferable for different interviewers to see the two groups so that there is no danger of an accidental breach of confidentiality. It also ensures that the two sets of data are not contaminated by any bias from interviewers' perceptions, expectations or memories.

Another difficult ethical situation for interviewers arises when they feel that informants are in need of medical or social help. Should the interviewer attempt to intervene in any way? In my view it is appropriate for the interviewer to advise the person where or from whom they might get help and to give them names, addresses and telephone numbers. I think interviewers should offer to get in touch with the potential helper only at the informant's request, and should never do so without the informant's explicit agreement.

It may be somewhat inappropriate to describe the issues relating to the **contents of the questionnaire** as ethical, since they raise humanitarian rather than moral questions. Is it reasonable to ask people about things that they find painful or embarrassing? This again is not, I think, something that can be answered by a yes or no. Partly it depends on how it is done. If things are placed in a relevant context then people may find it acceptable to discuss issues that in other circumstances they would find distressing or embarrassing. Another factor to be taken into account is whether or not people will have had to confront the painful topic directly or whether it is something that they have been, and are, avoiding. If someone is bereaved – by the death of a relative, a still birth or by the loss of a job or a home – then they must have accepted it at one level or another. It may be painful to talk about, to relive the unhappiness, but it may also be helpful to do so. Indeed one of the problems faced by bereaved people is that friends and relatives are sometimes unwilling to let them talk about it and to let them grieve; for these people the opportunity to talk may be almost therapeutic. It is likely to be more helpful if they are given an opportunity to express their feelings rather than be restricted by rigid adherence to a structured questionnaire and the use of pre-coded questions. But while bereavement must be recognised, future bereavements, although inevitable, may not. It then becomes questionable whether surveys should open up such topics, and to what extent it is reasonable to pursue them. The question of whether people with a terminal illness knew that they were dying was discussed earlier. Another subject likely to be painful is how parents of handicapped children feel about the survival of the children. Direct questions might be almost cruel, but an opportunity to discuss their feelings with a non-directive and skilled interviewer who is felt to be sympathetic would probably reveal whether parents now feel it would have been better if the child had not survived.

The potential embarrassment of informants is another possibility that has to be faced in drawing up a questionnaire. The problem needs to be considered in relation to response rates and the need not to alienate either informants or interviewers. What people find embarrassing obviously changes over time. Earlier, I discussed how at one stage OPCS felt it was inappropriate to ask single women about their use of contraception, but were prepared to do so within a relatively short time. I think embarrassment is infectious and it is important to ensure that interviewers are not embarrassed by the questions they have to ask. Now it is commonly held that more people are reluctant to respond to questions about income than to those about contraception or sex. But reactions to questions about income may more usually be described as resentment about prying than as embarrassment. If the majority of people are prepared to answer such questions it seems reasonable to include them, but if many do not wish to do so it is foolhardy, rather than immoral or unkind, to ask them – and in that situation the quality of the data obtained is likely to be unsatisfactory.

Confidentiality has to be safeguarded in the **data processing** of survey data. Analysis by computer seems to give rise to particular concern. But for the most part survey information that is put on to a computer, or indeed on to punched cards, cannot be related to individuals without reference to lists or records linking names with serial numbers. It is the confidentiality of these lists or records that needs to be safeguarded. Using serial numbers on questionnaires without names helps to preserve confidentiality, but of course does not guarantee it.

Names, and other characteristics of identity such as dates of birth and addresses, may be used in the processing if survey data are to be linked with information from other records, and it is in this situation that particular vigilance is needed to safeguard confidentiality.

Confidentiality is also one of the main ethical issues involved in the **presentation of results**. There are normally no problems with statistical presentations, but with illustrative data identities may need to be disguised even though no names are mentioned. How far should confidentiality be extended to institutions as well as individuals? If patients criticise or praise specific hospitals or clinics, should they be identified? And do the same criteria apply to professionals as to patients? In practice there are rarely any problems but in theory I think the question of confidentiality in relation to professionals could present difficulties if a survey revealed evidence of ill treatment, negligence or incompetence. For example, what would be the position if a court called for interview data to be presented as evidence?

On a lighter note, when people refuse to be interviewed no guarantees of confidentiality have normally been given. In our study of abortion patients (Cartwright and Lucas 1974) we considered identifying the hospitals and the clinics who refused to participate. I do not think that that would have been unethical.

The other ethical issue in the presentation of results relates to the suppression of information. In broad terms it seems unethical on the part of either the researcher, or the person or organisation sponsoring the research, to suppress statistical findings relating to health and health care. Some funding bodies, such as the DHSS, make it a condition that they should receive a copy of any paper before it is submitted for publication. Any comments from the Department received within 28 days should be considered by the author but it is not intended that this should restrict in any way a researcher's right to freely publish the results. However, if a researcher hopes to obtain further funding from the Department it is almost inevitable that some constraints will be felt. It is certainly advisable that researchers and funders should define and agree their rights and powers over this from the start. And some researchers in the health field may well feel it is unethical to undertake work without a clear agreement that any results may be published.

Use of surveys

Obviously the way a survey is used – and the extent to which it is used – depends on its aims, procedures and results, but its use is also related to who funds it, who does it, the timing, and the way the results are presented and disseminated. So the use of surveys is discussed in relation to these characteristics before looking at the impact and contribution of survey results.

Initiation and funding The main funders of surveys in the health and health care fields are government – the Department of Health and Social Security, Scottish Home and Health Department, Office of Population Censuses and Surveys, and Local Health Authorities; research councils – the Medical Research Council and the Social Science Research Council; research foundations, such as the Nuffield Provincial Hospitals Trust, King's Fund, Rowntree Trust, Ford Foundation, Leverhulme Trust; organisations with specific research or educational interests such as the Health Education Council, the Cancer Research Campaign, the National Fund for Research into Crippling Diseases; universities; commercial organisations such as the pharmaceutical industry and the British United Provident Association; and the media – television and the press.

Nearly all these bodies may initiate surveys, and so too may pressure groups and independent research institutes, but the distribution of funders and initiators is very different and the person or organisation who initiated a study is more difficult to identify. Rothschild in his discussion of the organisation and management of government research and development (1971) saw the funder as the initiator: research 'with a practical application as its objective, must be done on a customer-contractor* basis: the customer says what he wants; the contractor does it (if he can); and the customer pays'. In practice, the relationships between the initiator, the funder and the researcher, particularly for government supported research, is more complicated. As McKeown (1973) has put it, 'the interests of the customer and contractor should be merged to enable the customer to have the advice and assistance of the contractor, and to give the contractor the interest and incentive to modify or enlarge his research interests'.

If an organisation has funded a survey it will normally take some interest in the results and at least will be aware of the study. So surveys funded by government departments might be expected to make the most impact in terms of influencing policy. But there are a number of reasons why surveys that are both initiated and funded by government departments may not be so influential in that sort of way:

1 They are unlikely to question basic government policy.

* The 'customer' is the funder, the 'contractor' the researcher.

2 They are likely to be directed at the immediate, day to day problems of administrators.

3 The production of data may be seen as the end result: resources for analysis may not be forthcoming, comment on findings may be discouraged and comparisons with other studies seen as irrelevant.

4 Surveys may sometimes be initiated in order to postpone actions or decisions, and be presented as an alternative to action.

5 Changes in government or in civil service personnel may mean that the person who initiated the survey and might have been keen to take action on the basis of the results may no longer be in a position to do so when the results become available.

Research councils and universities are the organisations most willing to sponsor academic research with theoretical rather than practical objectives, and surveys initiated by universities are probably the most esoteric and the most radical. There is also the danger that surveys initiated by universities are liable to become overloaded by different theories, imaginative explanations and academic curiosity.

Government departments, universities and research councils are all concerned to some extent with academic respectability, but government departments are most likely to want surveys based on nationally representative samples. Both government and research councils have fairly elaborate structures for research management to evaluate not only the quality of research proposals but also their potential value. However, the criteria on which they assess this is, as has already been discussed, rather different – government departments looking for surveys with relatively practical, immediate and basically conservative implications, research councils placing more emphasis on theory.

Research foundations and organisations with specific interests vary from the relatively academic to the frankly partisan. I do not think there can be much doubt that pressure groups use their research to further their own ends: supporting surveys likely to substantiate their viewpoint and emphasising that part of the results which does so most clearly. Pressure groups are likely to be concerned with academic respectability mainly in so far as it affects their credibility and acceptability. Other organisations with specific interests may view surveys as an appropriate part of their activities but they may have little skill in formulating or recognising the questions that surveys can reasonably answer and see surveys about their interest as a way of furthering that interest without any clear understanding of the way in which they might do so.

Finally, commercial organisations and the media may promote surveys likely to produce results of a particular nature. The media want dramatic news; the commercial organisation an outcome that in one way or another will make it more profitable. Their interests inevitably affect the content and the use of the surveys they are willing to support.

This may sound cynical but I have aimed at identifying relevant interests and potential dangers. What actually happens depends on the response and initiative of the organisations who carry out surveys.

Survey organisations Government, research councils, and universities are all in the business of doing health surveys, so too are a number of independent and commercial organisations, the media and quite a few practitioners in the health field. The ways they initiate and respond to requests for surveys, conduct the studies and disseminate the results determine the usefulness of surveys and the way they are used. To illustrate the variety in the type of response and activity, I propose to discuss briefly the use and type of health surveys most often carried out by the Government Social Survey, by university departments and by the media.

The Government Social Survey is funded by government and does surveys that are initiated by government departments. In theory it does not initiate studies itself; in practice there are opportunities to exert at least some influence on government departments in their requests. Because of the way it is funded and its studies are initiated, its surveys are exposed to the dangers listed earlier (pages 186–187). I think it is a tribute to its management and staff that in the main they have succeeded in resisting these pressures. Inevitably there have been, and are, problems. I regard the General Household Survey as overloaded and inadequately analysed. Some of the other GSS studies described in this review (Gregory, 1978, Ritchie, Jacoby and Bone 1978) appear to ignore other relevant research. I am not critical so much of the authors but of the system which puts pressure on them to produce statistics and reports but does not allow adequate time for literature research or for analysing and discussing the results. But technically, GSS surveys are highly competent: its samples are well designed and its interviewers highly trained. In some ways its organisation seems lopsided: it collects good and reliable data but could do more with them.

University departments mainly do research that has been initiated by academics, including academic practitioners. The surveys are generally local rather than national. There is an academic orientation, particularly in departments without clinical responsibilities, so surveys are usually placed in a theoretical framework and related to other studies in the field. The audience to which the survey publications are addressed is often other academics in the same field, and this in my view is the most severe limitation on the use of health surveys carried out in university departments of sociology. Because of the other commitments of the academics involved, surveys done in this setting tend to have a relatively long time scale which can also affect their usefulness. For tenured academics there is little pressure to adhere to intended deadlines for reports. Indeed the academic atmosphere and ethos run almost counter to the notion that such deadlines are appropriate.

On the other hand it is from university departments that the thoughtful analysis of underlying implications is likely to emerge. Titmuss's study of the gift relationship involved in donating blood (page 122) will probably be remembered and quoted when the surveys done by government departments are gathering dust in the attics or cellars of libraries. And it is in university departments and independent research units that the more radical surveys are likely to be done.

Media research is sure of publicity, but is it used? Its impact is probably transitory, and its message may be recognised but rejected with relative ease by those who find it unpalatable on the grounds that its methods were unscientific. At the same time it has the enormous advantage that it is done quickly and its timing is right: it is nearly always published when interest in the subject is high – because that was the reason for doing the research in the first place.

Timing Since studies tend to be initiated and planned when there is particular interest in the subject, the speed with which a survey is carried out is likely to affect its topicality. The real skill is in selecting topics that *will* be of concern by the time the survey is ready for publication. Media concern leads to publicity and this can influence the extent to which a survey is noticed and used. Fortuitous events can affect the impact of a survey greatly. The fieldwork of Shepperdson's study of two groups of parents with Down's syndrome children (page 82) had been completed when a pediatrician, Dr Leonard Arthur, was charged with the murder of a baby with Down's syndrome. *The Times* heard about the research and did a short article on it (21 8 81). A letter based on the article was subsequently published in the *Lancet* (Simms 1981) and this in turn was quoted by counsel at the trial of Dr Arthur.

I quote this to illustrate that research findings emerging at a time when the results are particularly apposite are likely to be extensively used, although they may be misunderstood. *The Times* report put considerable emphasis on a difference which, when Shepperdson herself produced a report for publication, turned out not to be statistically significant. But some researchers might prefer misquotation to the oblivion to which survey reports can be assigned if they do not appear at a pertinent time.

Another common problem is for clinicians and administrators to discount critical findings of a survey on the grounds that they are out of date.

Presentation and dissemination of results The results of the surveys discussed in this review have been published in a wide range of forms, from *Woman's Own* to the *Lancet*, in long, library-only type books (Kohn and White 1976) as well as popular paperback (Boyd and Sellers 1982) and the 'reference-rather-than-read' series of the General Household Survey. The form of publication is influenced by the audience to which it is addressed or to whom it is likely to appeal; the concentration of aims (surveys with fairly diffuse aims tend to be reported in books, those with single objectives in journals) and the nature of the material to be presented. These three considerations can produce conflicts. A researcher may wish to address a wide audience but feel, as I do, that the evidence should be made available for people to assess the validity of the conclusions and it is difficult to present much statistical material in a popular report. An obvious solution is to present the material in more than one form, addressed to different audiences: scientific and popular. Another is to present the material in a scientific form and then publicise and disseminate results through newspaper articles and reviews, in talks to the public, professionals and pressure groups, at seminars and meetings, or on the radio or television. The media can be courted. Some researchers do this assiduously, others shun the media and fight shy of presenting their material in different forms. This seems to me to be one reason why survey results are not used or recognised as widely as they might be.

There are several reasons why survey researchers in the health field do not devote more time and skill to presenting results in different forms so that they reach wider and appropriate audiences. An obvious one is *time*. A number of the people doing surveys in the health field are teachers and clinicians with other commitments and demands on their time. But even full-time researchers are often being urged to undertake further research rather than spend more time presenting results from earlier studies in different ways. Sometimes people under-estimate the time it takes to analyse and write up results once they have been collected. (The most frequent comment I make on grant applications is that insufficient time has been allowed for this.) In addition full-time researchers often need to obtain funding and support for their next project while they are writing the report on their current project. This diverts their energies and enthusiasm and uses up time. *The way much health research is funded* also discourages additional publications because few research staff have permanent appointments. Junior staff in particular are likely to change jobs at the end of a project. And being involved in a new project or another type of job inevitably dilutes their capacity and their will to spend time on an old one. Essentially a 'dissemination phase' needs to be funded as part of the basic project (see Gordon and Meadows 1981).

Another reason is *inclination*. Many researchers find it tedious and even somewhat depressing to devote time to presenting material in different ways. They tend to be concerned with the problems at which the research was directed, stimulated by the challenge of designing an appropriate project, excited by unravelling the results but bored by reworking them. They may dislike giving talks or being interviewed and they may not be particularly good at doing these things. So *lack of skill* is another problem; researchers do not necessarily possess the ability to present their data in exciting ways or in different forms.

In addition *motivation* is often lacking. Having written up results in one form they have fulfilled their obligations. There is little or no encouragement or pressure to do more. Their careers and reputations depend on academic rather than popular publications. They may be inclined to regard journals and magazines with a wide circulation but an unscholarly presentation or activist approach as second rate. And funders demanding a lengthy and detailed report which is not suitable for publication is an added disincentive to the production of yet more reports. Fortunately in this country we do not assess a researcher simply by the number of publications.

Finally, there is the question of *ignorance*: researchers may be unaware of the potential audience for their findings.

So, for these various reasons, I doubt if many premenopausal women are aware of the few symptoms they are likely to experience when they reach menopause; whether many organisers of health services are aware of the widespread prevalence of foot problems;

whether many general practitioners realise that they might reduce their consultation rates by distributing a simple booklet about six common symptoms suffered by children, or that some groups of their patients may not 'cash' two-fifths of their prescriptions. But of course results of some surveys are known, but not acted on.

Impact and contribution of survey results To take an extreme example first: almost everyone now knows that smoking is associated with lung cancer, most accept that the relationship is causal but while cigarette smoking has declined among doctors and there has been some drop in the cigarette consumption of men, that of women has increased substantially since Doll and Hill published their findings. In addition, regular cigarette smoking is starting at an increasingly earlier age (Todd 1975). Anxiety and guilt among smokers has probably risen as a result of these studies which, on the basis of these changes, might appear to have had relatively little impact and not all of that good. It might have been hoped that most smokers would have given it up and that virtually no one would have started. But it is impossible to know what would have happened if the relationship between lung cancer and smoking had not been identified. Smoking levels might now be appreciably higher and no attempt would have been made to identify and remove carcinogenic agents in tobacco. The demands of non-smokers for non-smoking areas in aeroplanes, cinemas and restaurants might have gone unheeded, while general attitudes to smoking and smokers might be very different. Certainly the results had an impact on a wide range of people: smokers and non-smokers, doctors, teachers, the tobacco industry, the retail trade, the media, the advertising industry and the government. But even in such a clear-cut study it is impossible to identify the precise nature and extent of the impact.

Some survey results seem to make little or no impact. As Macintyre (1981) has pointed out, surveys have produced evidence of long waiting times and unsatisfactory conditions at ante-natal clinics over many decades but they still persist. The impact of a survey is probably influenced by the way it is presented, the timing, the funder and by the organisation or individuals doing it. It may also be affected by the quality of the survey but this is by no means certain. It may be difficult to ignore the results of large scale, national surveys but people may be stimulated to action more often by surveys on their doorstep: it may be easier for local surveys to lead to local change than for national ones to affect national policy or practice.

In my view the surveys most likely to make an obvious and effective impact are those taken up by pressure groups or done in fields where change was imminent anyway and only the precise form and nature of the change uncertain. An evaluation of stroke units is likely to make an impact if a new hospital is being planned or hospital services for an area are under review. A survey of patients' views and experiences of mixed wards is likely to be taken into account if mixed wards are being considered. At the same time I feel that the main contribution that surveys make is to scientific knowledge and to the somewhat nebulous 'climate of opinion'. I would postulate that surveys of patients' experiences and views have influenced attitudes of professionals, but I would be hard put to produce clear evidence of that.

Bulmer (1982) emphasises a rather different role for social research. Summarising recent, mainly American, studies of policy and decision making in government he concludes: 'Research provides the intellectual background of concepts, orientations and empirical generalisations that inform policy. It is used to orient decision-makers to problems, to think about and specify the problematic elements in a situation, to get new ideas. Policy-makers use research to formulate problems and to set the agenda for future policy actions. Much of this use is not direct, but a result of long-term infiltration of social science concepts, theories and findings with the general intellectual culture of a society' (page 48 of study). He quotes Weiss (1977) as drawing the conclusion that: 'There is a role for research as social criticism . . . As new concepts and data emerge, their gradual cumulative effect can be to change the conventions policy makers abide by and to reorder the goals and priorities of policy makers.' Many of the surveys discussed in this review have more practical and limited implications, but nevertheless they have probably been influential in widening the horizons of policy makers and making them rethink comfortable assumptions.

Potential of health and health care surveys

Since surveys are initiated, funded and carried out by a wide variety of organisations with different concerns and capabilities, it is not surprising if the distribution of topics covered in surveys is not, in sum, particularly rational or even. Some areas may attract researchers or funders because they are academically acceptable, or political appealing, or of direct concern to their interests, or demand particular techniques, or are likely to come up with newsworthy results. In this situation it is almost inevitable that some fields are over surveyed and others neglected.

Since this review is far from comprehensive it cannot attempt any systematic assessment of gaps. Nevertheless I think it has identified some subject areas that are under-explored and some methods that are under-used. To take the under-used methods first, there seem to be eight **techniques or approaches that could usefully be used more often**:

1 **Postal inquiries** These have tended to be used for surveys of professionals and to identify samples with particular character- istics. Evaluation had been largely concerned with response rates and with identifying possible bias in response. Good response rates can be obtained to relatively long questionnaires if they are addressed to people with some interest in and commitment to the subject. This was so for the survey of patients who had been in hospital and, more recently, for a study of infant feeding (Martin and Monk 1982). What needs now to be evaluated is the accuracy and repeat- ability of such responses and how that compares with information ob- tained by interviews or from records. Postal studies are not only rela- tively cheap, they have the advantage of not needing to be cluster- ed geographically and therefore have smaller sampling errors.

2 **Telephone interviews** are another possibility, but since only three quarters of households have the use of a telephone (Office of Population Censuses and Surveys 1982b) this approach can only be used in conjuction with interviews or postal inquiries among those without a telephone. Again it would be necessary to compare and evaluate the responses obtained by different techniques.

3 **Diaries or log books** These have been used on a number of studies discussed in this review (see pages 74, 90, 129). It is a useful technique and probably improves the quality of data collected. I think it could be used more often. For instance, certain patients might be asked to keep a diary of selected symptoms after they have been discharged from hospital. If the diaries were mailed to the hospital they could be scanned to identify particular problems and then filed in records for future reference. Log books might also be used to check drug consumption and adherence to important regimes; a recent study assessed outcomes of different methods of treatment by getting women to keep a pain diary (Pearce, Knight

and Beard 1982). As has been shown, diaries can be used to give a picture of the way professional resources are used. I have identified other ways in which they might also be used, but these uses would need to be validated initially.

4 **Validation of results** Sometimes the only way to do this is by a second survey, a technique employed in a number of health fields, but not in others. This was discussed on page 175. Another validation technique is by comparison with data obtained in other ways; this too has been inadequately exploited. For example, many of the health data collected in the General Household Survey need to be validated by specific studies. Lack of validation leads to surveys being disregarded and dismissed as 'soft' data.

5 **Use of different sampling frames** National sampling frames of births, deaths, marriages and divorces have rarely, if at all, been used for health surveys. It may seem to be putting things back to front to suggest a possible sample without discussing the subject matter of formulating specific questions. But I would argue that considering what can be done with a sample can suggest questions that can be usefully answered. (I confess that the idea for the study of the needs of the dying (pages 47–48) arose after I had done a study based on the registration of births which made me think about other available sampling frames.)

6 **Follow-up studies** of people receiving medical or other forms of health care. Because this approach does not involve comparisons or specific hypotheses I think it has been undervalued – and therefore under-used. I hope that pages 79–84 have illustrated its usefulness. To fully exploit it we need to *develop better indices of the quality of life*.

7 **Repeated surveys over time in a single population** The UK has the three national birth cohort studies in which children have been surveyed at different stages of development, but there has been no geographical area in which the population has been repeatedly surveyed. Yet such an approach can illuminate the natural history of disease, as in the Framingham study in America which was concerned with the epidemiology of arterosclerotic disease (Dawber 1980); and the Alameda County studies which related various health practices to physical health status (Belloc and Breslow 1972); and to mortality (Breslow and Enstram 1980). This last study also showed that social networks were related to mortality independently of a number of factors including smoking habits, alcohol

consumption, physical activity and the use of preventive health services (Berkman and Syme 1979).

8 **Opportunistic studies exploiting sudden and unexpected changes** One such study used the opportunity of a hospital strike to look at maternal attitudes to unintended home confinements. It seems likely that we may have the chance to look at the effects of further strikes and the consequent postponement, and sometimes the complete cancellation, of some planned interventions. A problem in this situation is raising money and finding facilities quickly enough.

Turning to the **subject areas that are under-explored**, a number of specific gaps have been suggested by this review.

One is the effects and side effects of care or treatment. Many types of surgical, medical and paramedical intervention have not been exposed to follow-up studies or adequate assessment of their effects on patients' lives. Indeed, many treatments have become firmly established without having been critically evaluated. Another gap is that clinical effects are often evaluated but the social effects ignored. I would like to see more surveys of patients' experience and views carried out in conjunction with clinical trials.

Initially, surveys in the health field were dominated by medical models and this is still a weakness of some of the work being done. Clinicians are interested in patients' compliance, and one study (pages 92–93) demonstrated the importance of assessing patients' adherence to drug or, indeed, any other regimen when carrying out clinical trials. But adherence to medical advice or prescription ought to be studied in a wider context and related to doctors' intentions when giving the advice and to the reasons why patients do not follow it. Surveys tend to look at subjects from the point of view of either the patients or the health professionals when it would be more illuminating to look at the links between the two – and to ask how the views and experiences of patients and professionals relate to one another. This is particularly true of studies of the organisation of health care – a field to which surveys could usefully contribute more. For instance, continuity of care from general practitioners is a concept which is much debated but few systematic studies of its implications for patients and for doctors have been carried out. And the scope for exploring the implications of different organisational procedures in hospital by systematic surveys is so under-used as to suggest the existence of powerful and almost impenetrable barriers.

Surveys can also contribute to the cost-benefit analysis of different forms of health care. Their particular function in this field is to ensure that the needs of patients for tender loving care are given due consideration. On the organisational side I am less certain whether surveys can show us how to translate these needs into action, but they could in theory be used to demonstrate some of the ways in which the dominance and power of various interest groups operate.

The collection of routine statistics and returns made by health professionals, another organisational matter, could sometimes be replaced by ad hoc or regular surveys. In some circumstances surveys might be a more useful, economic and accurate way to collect data: they might answer more of the relevant questions, more directly and more accurately. They would generally cause less work and frustration for the people involved in providing the service and enable them to spend more time on their basic professional jobs. And survey data are seldom completely unanalysed or ignored in the way that some routine returns seem to be.

Other topics inadequately covered by surveys are common health problems which tend not to appeal to either sponsors or researchers as much as new and rare ones. This is partly because there may not be any new ideas to explore in relation to, say, coughs, colds, backache or bunions, but I think another reason is that the common problems are less newsworthy and less prestigious. That I suspect is one reason why the survey on trouble with feet has never been followed up or replicated: to study feet is somehow ignominious.

Another neglected area, this time partly for technical reasons, is in the needs of, and services for, people with communication problems – people who are deaf, confused or with speech difficulties. There are some exceptions and some researchers have devised ingenious techniques to try to overcome the problems (Willocks, Cook, Ring and Kelleher 1980).

These gaps suggest that surveys could have something of an elitist effect, concentrating attention on esoteric conditions and articulate patients, away from common problems and the more deprived patients. Also, I have argued that most of the surveys on acceptability have somewhat conservative implications: they may indicate ways in which existing services might be modified but cannot explore potentialities of new services. In spite of these limitations, however, I think that surveys in the health field generally have a radical, but not a revolutionary, impact. Surveys revealing variations in care have radical implications while those concerned with health professionals can identify need for reforms (for example, suggest a more adequate training of medical students in contraception).

But the most fundamental contribution made by surveys in the health field is that most of them are concerned with the needs, experiences and attitudes of patients in a service which might otherwise be dominated by professional paternalism. In a very real sense, surveys are part of a democratic process: they are essentially sample referendums. For the most part they are concerned with the humanitarianism of health services, but they can also shed some light on clinical competence and organisational efficiency. In addition, they can illuminate unmet needs, reveal inappropriate use of services, identify effects of care, and highlight inequalities in the distribution of services, care and needs.

References

Alderson, M R, and Dowie, Robin (1979) Health surveys and related studies. Oxford: Pergamon Press.

Allen, Isobel (1982) Short-stay residential care for the elderly. London: Policy Studies Institute.

Anderson J A D; Buck, Carol; Danaher, Kate and Fry, John (1977) 'Users and non-users of doctors – implications for self-care' Journal of the Royal College of General Practitioners 27 155–159.

Anderson, J E; Morrell, D C; Avery A J and Watkins, C J (1980) 'Evaluation of a patient education manual' British Medical Journal 281 924–926.

Arber, Sara and Sawyer, Lucianne (1981) 'Changes in general practice: do patients benefit?' British Medical Journal 283 1367–1370.

Ashley, J S A Personal communication.

Ashley, J S A; Howlett, Ann and Morris, J N (1971) 'Case-fatality of hyperplasia of the prostate in two teaching and three regional-board hospitals' Lancet 2 1308–1311.

Atkinson, Jean (1971) A handbook for interviewers. OPCS Social Survey Division. London: HMSO.

Austin, Pam; Lewis, Denis and Scammell, Brian (1977) A review of postal surveys. OPCS Methodology Series Paper – draft.

Baker, C D (1976) 'Non-attenders in general practice' Journal of the Royal College of General Practitioners 26 404–409.

Beaumont, Berenice (1978) 'Training and careers of women doctors in the Thames regions' British Medical Journal 1 191–193.

Beaumont, Berenice (1979) 'Special provisions for women doctors to train and practise in medicine after graduation: a report of a survey' Medical Education 13 284–291.

Beer, T C; Goldenberg, E; Smith, D S and Mason, A S (1974) 'Can I have an ambulance doctor?' British Medical Journal 1 226–228.

Belloc, Nedra B and Breslow, Lester (1972) 'Relationship of physical health status and health practices' Preventive Medicine 1 409–421.

Bennett, A E; Garrad, Jessie and Halil, T (1970) 'Chronic disease and disability in the community: a prevalence study' British Medical Journal iii 762–764.

Beresford, S A A; Chant, A D B; Jones, H O; Piachaud, D and Weddell, J M (1978) 'Varicose veins: a comparison of surgery and injection/compression sclerotherapy' Lancet 1 921–924.

Berkman, Lisa F and Syme, S Leonard (1979) 'Social networks, host resistance and mortality: a nine year follow up study of Alameda County residents' American Journal of Epidemiology 109 186–204.

Bevan, J M and Draper, G J (1967) Appointment systems in general practice. London: Oxford University Press.

Blaxter, Mildred (1976) The meaning of disability. London: Heinemann.

Blaxter, Mildred (1981) The health of children: a review of research on the place of health in cycles of disadvantage. London: Heinemann.

Blaxter, Mildred and Paterson, Elizabeth (1982) Mothers and daughters: a three generational study of health attitudes and behaviour. London: Heinemann Educational Books.

Blomfield, J M and Douglas, J W B (1956) 'Bedwetting: prevalence among children aged 4–7 years' Lancet 1 850–852.

Blyth, W G and Marchant, L J (1973) 'A self-weighting random sampling technique' Journal of Market Research Society 15 157–163.

Bone, Margaret (1973) Family planning services in England and Wales. London: HMSO.

Bone, Margaret (1978) The family planning services: changes and effects. London: HMSO.

Bonnar, John; Goldberg, A and Smith, Jacqueline A (1969) 'Do pregnant women take their iron?' Lancet 1 457–458.

Bowling, Ann and Cartwright, Ann (1982) Life after a death. London: Tavistock.

Boyd, Catherine and Sellers, Lea (1982) The British way of birth. London: Pan Books.

Bradshaw, J (1972) 'A taxonomy of social need' In Problems and progress in medical care: essays on current research. Seventh series. Edited by G. McLachlan. Oxford University Press for Nuffield Provincial Hospitals Trust.

Breslow, Lester and Enstrom, James E (1980) 'Persistence of health habits and their relationship to mortality' Preventive Medicine 9 469–483.

Brewer, Colin (1977) 'Third time unlucky: a study of women who have three or more legal abortions' Journal of Biosocial Science 9 99–105.

British Medical Journal (1946) 'Are the people more healthy?' 1 318–319.

British Medical Journal (1952) 'Smoking and lung cancer' 2 1299–1301.

British Medical Journal (1954) 'Lung cancer and smoking' 1 445–465.

British Medical Journal (1957) 'Dangers of cigarette smoking' 1 1518–1520.

British Medical Journal (1964) 'Deaths from smoking' 2 1451–1452.

British Medical Journal (1979) 'Non-compliance: does it matter?' 2 1168.

British Medical Journal (1980) 'Junior doctors' work load. Results of BMA survey' 280 1632.

Brotherston, Sir John (Ed) (1978) Morbidity and its relationship to resource allocation. Welsh Office.

Buchan, I C and Richardson, I M (1973) Time study of consultations in general practice. Scottish Health Service Studies No. 27. Scottish Home and Health Department.

Bulman, J S; Richards, N D; Slack, G L and Willcocks, A J (1968) Demand and need for dental care. London: OUP.

Bulmer, Martin (1982) The uses of social research: social investigation in public policy-making. London: Allen and Unwin.

Bungay, G T; Vessey, M P and McPherson, C K (1980) 'Study of symptoms in middle life with special reference to the menopause' British Medical Journal 281 181–183.

Butler, J R (1980) How many patients?: a study of list sizes in general practice. Occasional Papers on Social Administration 64. London: Bedford Square Press.

Butler, J R; Bevan, J M and Taylor, R C (1973) Family doctors and public policy. London: Routledge and Kegan Paul.

Butler, J R and Knight, R (1975) 'Designated areas: a review of problems and policies' British Medical Journal 2 571–573.

Butler, N R and Alberman, E D (1969) Perinatal problems – the second report of the 1958 British perinatal mortality survey. Edinburgh: Livingstone.

Butler, N R and Bonham, D G (1963) Perinatal mortality: First report of the British perinatal mortality survey. Edinburgh: Livingstone.

Butler, N R; Goldstein, H and Ross, E M (1972) 'Cigarette smoking in pregnancy: its influence on birth weight and perinatal mortality' British Medical Journal 2 127–130.

Calnan, M; Douglas, J W B and Goldstein, H (1978) 'Tonsillectomy and circumcision: comparisons of two cohorts' International Journal of Epidemiology 7 79–85.

Cannell, Charles F; Marquis, Kent H and Laurent, André (1977) A summary of studies of interviewing methodology. Vital and Health Statistics Series 2 No. 69. Washington: PHS.

Carstairs, V and Morrison, M (1971) The elderly in residential care. Scottish Health Service Studies No. 19. Scottish Home and Health Department.

Cartwright, Ann (1959a) 'Some problems in the collection and analysis of morbidity data obtained from sample surveys' Milkbank Memorial Fund Quarterly 37 33–48.

Cartwright, Ann (1959b) 'The families and individuals who did not co-operate in a sample survey' Milbank Memorial Quarterly 37 347–368.

Cartwright, Ann (1964) Human relations and hospital care. London: Routledge and Kegan Paul.

Cartwright, Ann (1967) Patients and their doctors. London: Routledge and Kegan Paul.

Cartwright, Ann (1970) Parents and family planning services. London: Routledge and Kegan Paul.

Cartwright, Ann (1978) 'Professionals as responders: variations in and effects of response rates to questionnaires 1961–77' British Medical Journal 2 1419–1421.

Cartwright, Ann (1979) The dignity of labour? A study of childbearing and induction. London: Tavistock.

Cartwright, Ann and Anderson, Robert (1981) General practice revisited: a second study of patients and their doctors. London: Tavistock.

Cartwright, Ann, Hockey, L and Anderson, J L (1973) Life before death. London: Routledge and Kegan Paul.

Cartwright, Ann and Lucas, Susan (1974) 'Survey of abortion patients' Report of the Committee on the Working of the Abortion Act Vol. III. London: HMSO.

Cartwright, Ann; Lucas, Susan and O'Brien, Maureen (1976) 'Some methodological problems in studying consultations in general practice' Journal of the Royal College of General Practitioners 26 894–906.

Cartwright, Ann; Martin, F M and Thomson, J G (1959) 'Community aspects of a mass radiography campaign' Medical Officer 101 313–317.

Cartwright, Ann and O'Brien, Maureen (1976) 'Social class variations in health care and in the nature of general practitioner consultations.' In The Sociology of the NHS, edited by Margaret Stacey, Sociological Review Monograph No. 22.

Cartwright, Ann and Tucker, Wyn (1969) 'An experiment with an advance letter on an interview inquiry' British Journal of Preventive and Social Medicine 23 241–243.

Cartwright, Ann and Ward, Audrey W M (1968) 'Variations in general practitioners' response to postal questionnaires' British Journal of Preventive and Social Medicine 22 199–205.

Central Statistical Office (1975) 'Social commentary: social class' In Social Trends No. 6., CSO. London: HMSO.

Chamberlain, Geoffrey; Philipp, Elliot; Howlett, Brian and Masters, Keith (1978) British Births 1970 Vol. 2. Obstetric Care London: Heinemann Medical.

Chamberlain, Roma; Chamberlain, Geoffrey; Howlett, Brian and Claireaux, Albert (1975) British Births 1970 Vol. 1. The first week of life. London: Heinemann Medical.

Chant, A D B; Jones, H O and Weddell, J M (1972) 'Varicose veins: a comparison of surgery and injection/compression sclerotherapy' Lancet 2 1188–1191.

Clarke, May (1969) Trouble with feet. Occasional Papers on Social Administration No. 29. London: G. Bell & Sons Ltd.

Clarke, May (1978) 'Getting through the work' in Readings in the sociology of nursing edited by Robert Dingwall and Jean Macintosh. London: Churchill Livingstone.

Cochrane, A L (1954) 'Detection of pulmonary tuberculosis in a community' British Medical Bulletin 10 91–95.

Cochrane, A L (1972) Effectiveness and efficiency: random reflections on health services. London: Nuffield Provincial Hospitals Trust.

Colley, J R T; Douglas, J W B and Reid, D D (1973) 'Respiratory disease in young adults: influence of early childhood lower respiratory tract illness, social class, air pollution and smoking' British Medical Journal 2 195–198.

Collins, Elizabeth and Klein, Rudolf (1980) 'Equity and the NHS: self-reported morbidity, access and primary care' British Medical Journal 281 1111–1115.

Cooper, Peter; Gath, Dennis; Rose, Nicholas and Fieldsend, Robert (1982) 'Psychological sequelae to elective sterilisation: a prospective study' British Medical Journal 284 461–464.

Coronary Drug Project Research Group (1980) 'Influence of adherence to treatment and response of cholesterol on mortality in the coronary drug project' New England Journal of Medicine 303 1038–1041.

Cunningham, D J; Bevan, J M and Floyd, C B (1972) 'The role of the practice nurse from the patient's point of view' Community Medicine 128 534–538.

Davie, Ronald (1973) 'Eleven years of childhood' CSO Statistical News No. 22 14–18.

Davie, R; Butler, N and Goldstein, H (1972) From birth to seven. The second report of the National Child Development Study. London: Longman.

Dawber, Thomas Royle (1980) The Framingham Study: the epidemiology of atherosclerotic disease. London: Harvard University Press.

Department of Health and Social Security (1972) Enquiry into the previous medical experience of doctors joining the General Medical Services for the first time as unrestricted principals or as assistants (England & Wales). Reports on Health and Social Subjects No. 2. London: HMSO.

Department of Health and Social Security (1975) Review body on doctors' and dentists' remuneration. London: HMSO.

Department of Health and Social Security (1976) Sharing resources for health in England. Report of the Resource Allocation Working Party. London: HMSO.

Department of Health and Social Security (1978) Health Services Development: The provision of stoma care. H.C. 78.

Department of Health and Social Security. Research Working Group (1980) Inequalities in health: Report of a research working group. (Black Report) DHSS.

DerSimonian, Rebecca; Charette, Joseph; McPeek, Buckmann and Mosteller, Frederick (1982) 'Reporting on methods in clinical trials' New England Journal of Medicine 306 1332–1337.

Devlin, H Brendan; Plant, J A and Griffin, M (1971) 'Aftermath of surgery for anorectal cancer' British Medical Journal 3 413–418.

Doll, Richard and Hill, A Bradford (1950) 'Smoking and carcinoma of the lung preliminary report' British Medical Journal 2 739–748.

Doll, Richard and Hill, A Bradford (1952) 'A study of the aetiology of carcinoma of the lung' British Medical Journal 2 1271–1286.

Doll, Richard and Hill, A Bradford (1954) 'The mortality of doctors in relation to their smoking habits: a preliminary report' British Medical Journal 1 1451–1455.

Doll, Richard and Hill, A Bradford (1956) 'Lung cancer and other causes of death in relation to smoking: a second report on the mortality of British doctors' British Medical Journal 2 1071–1081.

Doll, Richard and Hill, A Bradford (1964) 'Mortality in relation to smoking: ten years' observations of British doctors' British Medical Journal 1 1399–1410, 1460–1467.

Douglas, J W B (1948) Maternity in Great Britain. A survey of social and economic aspects of pregnancy and childbirth London: OUP.

Douglas, J W B (1951) 'Social class differences in health and survival during the first two years of life; the results of a national survey' Population Studies 5 35–58.

Douglas, J W B (1956a) 'The age at which premature children walk' The Medical Officer 95 33–35.

Douglas, J W B (1956b) 'Mental ability and school achievement of premature children at 8 years of age' British Medical Journal 1 1210–1214.

Douglas, J W B (1964) The home and the school: A study of ability and attainment in the primary schools. London: MacGibbon & Kee.

Douglas, J W B (1976) 'The use and abuse of national cohorts' In The organisation and impact of social research edited by Marten Shipman. London: Routledge & Kegan Paul.

Douglas, J W B and Blomfield, J M (1956) 'The reliability of longitudinal studies' Milbank Memorial Fund Quarterly 34 227–252.

Douglas, J W B; Kiernan, K E and Wadsworth, M E J (1977) 'A longitudinal study of health and behaviour' Proceedings of the Royal Society of Medicine 70 530–532.

Douglas, J W B and Mogford, C (1953a) 'Health of premature children from birth to four years' British Medical Journal 1 748–754.

Douglas, J W B and Mogford, C (1953b) 'The results of a national inquiry into the growth of premature children from birth to 4 years' Archives of Disease in Childhood 28 436–445.

Douglas, J W B; Ross, J M and Simpson, H R (1968) All our future. London: Davies.

Douglas, J W B and Waller, R E (1966) 'Air pollution and respiratory infection in children' British Journal of Preventive and Social Medicine 20 1–8.

Dunnell, Karen (1979) Family formation 1976. London: HMSO.

Dunnell, Karen and Cartwright, Ann (1972) Medicine takers, prescribers and hoarders. London: Routledge and Kegan Paul.

Dunnell, Karen and Dobbs, Joy (1982) National survey of nurses working in the community. London: HMSO.

Earthrowl, B and Stacey, M (1977) 'Social class and children in hospital' Social Science and Medicine 11 83–88.

Ebrahim, S B J; Sainsbury, R and Watson, S (1981) 'Foot problems in the elderly: a hospital survey' British Medical Journal 283 949–950.

Exton-Smith, A N (1961) 'Terminal illness in the aged' Lancet 2 305–308.

Farrell, Christine (1978) My mother said . . . London: Routledge and Kegan Paul.

Fedrick, J; Alberman, E D and Goldstein, H (1971) 'Possible teratogenic effect of cigarette smoking' Nature 231 529–530.

Finch, Caroline (1981) 'General Household Survey letter experiments' Office of Population Censuses and Surveys Survey Methodology Bulletin No. 13.

Fisher, R A (1957a&b) 'Dangers of cigarette smoking' British Medical Journal 2 a) 43, b) 297–298.

Fisher, R A (1958a) 'Lung cancer and cigarettes?' Nature 182 108.

Fisher, R A (1958b) 'Cancer and smoking' Nature 182 596.

Fogelman, Ken (1976) Britain's sixteen-year-olds. London: National Children's Bureau.

Forster, D P (1976) 'Social class differences in sickness and general practice consultations' Health Trends 8 29–32.

Forster, D P (1978) 'Mortality as an indicator of morbidity in resource allocation' In Morbidity and its relationship to resource allocation edited by J H F Brotherston. Welsh Office.

Freeman, J and Byrne, P S (1976) 'The assessment of vocational training for general practice' Journal of the Royal College of General Practitioners. Reports from General Practice No. 17.

Freeman, J and Byrne, P S (1977) 'Clinical factual recall and patient management skill in general practice' Medical Education 11 39–47.

Fulton, Mary; Kellett, R J; Maclean, D W; Parkin, D M and Ryan, M P (1979) 'The management of hypertension – a survey of opinions among general practitioners' Journal of the Royal College of General Practitioners 29 583–587.

Garrad, Jessie and Bennett, A E (1971) 'A validated interview schedule for use in population surveys of chronic disease and disability' British Journal of Preventive and Social Medicine 25 97–104.

Garraway, W M; Akhtar, A J; Prescott, R J and Hockey, L (1980) 'Management of acute stroke in the elderly: preliminary results of a controlled trial' British Medical Journal 280 1040–1043.

Garraway, W M; Akhtar, A J; Hockey, L and Prescott, R J (1980) 'Management of acute stroke in the elderly: follow-up of a controlled trial' British Medical Journal 281 827–829.

Garraway, W M; Akhtar, A J; Smith, D L and Smith, M E (1981) 'The triage of stroke rehabilitation' Journal of Epidemiology and Community Health 35 39–44.

Garraway, W M; Walton, M S; Akhtar, A J and Prescott, R J (1981) 'The use of health and social services in the management of stroke in the community: results from a controlled trial. Age and Ageing 10 95–104.

Gilbert, G. Nigel; Arber, Sara and Dale, Angela (1980) 'SPSS and the General Household Survey' SSRC Survey Archive Bulletin, May.

Godber, Sir George (1981) 'Transatlantic contrasts in geriatrics' British Medical Journal 283 1326.

Golding, Jean (1979) Proposed design and estimated costs of a 4th National perinatal survey. Oxford: National Perinatal Epidemiology Unit.

Goldthorp, W O and Richman, J (1974) 'Maternal attitudes to unintended home confinement' The Practitioner 845–853.

Gordon, M D and Meadows, A J (1981) 'The dissemination of findings of DHSS-funded research' Primary Communications Research Centre, University of Leicester. ISBN 0 906083 18 4.

Graham, H (1978) Problems in antenatal care. University of York.

Gray, P G (1955) 'The memory factor in social surveys' Journal of the American Statistical Association 50 344–363.

Gray, P G and Corlett, T (1950) 'Sampling for the Social Survey' Journal of the Royal Statistical Society Series A 113 150–206.

Gray, P G and Gee, Frances A (1967) Electoral registration for parliamentary elections. London: HMSO.

Gray, P G, Corlett, T and Frankland, P (1956) 'The register of electors as a sampling frame.' In Readings in Market Research. London: British Market Research Bureau Ltd.

Gray, P G; Todd, J E; Slack, G L and Bulman, J S (1970) Adult dental health in England and Wales in 1968. London: HMSO.

Gregory, Janet (1978) Patients' attitudes to the hospital service: a survey carried out for the Royal Commission on the National Health Service. Research paper No. 5. London: HMSO.

Harris, Amelia I (1971) Handicapped and impaired in Great Britain, Part 1. London: HMSO.

Harris, Amelia I and Head, Elizabeth (1971 revised 1974) Sample surveys in local authority areas with particular reference to the handicapped and elderly. London: OPCS.

Hart, Julian Tudor (1970) 'Semi-continuous screening of a whole community for hypertension' Lancet 2 223–226.

Hart, Julian Tudor (1971) 'The inverse care law' Lancet 1 405–412.

Hart, Julian Tudor (1975) 'The management of high blood pressure in general practice' Journal of the Royal College of General Practitioners 25 160–192.

Hayman, Edward (1979) 'Interviewer coding of occupation and industry' Survey Methodology Bulletin No. 5. 12–14. OPCS.

Hinton, J (1980) 'Whom do dying patients tell?' British Medical Journal 281 1328–1330.

Hockey, Lisbeth (1966) Feeling the pulse. Queen's Institute of District Nursing.

Holohan, Ann M (1976) 'Accident and emergency departments: illness and accident behaviour' Sociological Review Monograph 22 111–119.

Holohan, Ann M; Newell, D J and Walker, J H (1975) 'Practitioners, patients and the accident department' Hospital and Health Services Review 71 80–84.

Hopkins, Anthony and Scambler, Graham (1977) 'How doctors deal with epilepsy' Lancet 1 183–186.

Hunt, Audrey (1970) The home help service in England and Wales. London: HMSO.

Hunt, Sonya M and McEwen, James (1980) 'The development of a subjective health indicator' Sociology of Health and Illness 2 231–246.

Hunt, Sonya M; McKenna, S P; McEwen, J; Backett, E M; Williams, Jan and Papp, Evelyn (1980) 'A quantitative approach to perceived health status: a validation study' Journal of Epidemiology and Community Health 34 281–286.

Hunt, Sonya M; McKenna, S P and Williams, Jan (1981) 'Reliability of a population survey tool for measuring perceived health problems: a study of patients with oseoarthritis' Journal of Epidemiology and Community Health 35 297–300.

Hunt, Sonya M; McKenna, S P; McEwan, J; Williams, Jan and Papp, Evelyn (1981) 'The Nottingham health profile: subjective health status and medical consultations' Social Science and Medicine 15A 221–229.

Illsley, R. (1956) 'The duration of antenatal care' Medical Officer 96 107–111.

Irvine, D and Jefferys, M (1971) 'BMA planning unit survey of general practice 1969' British Medical Journal 4 535–543.

Jacques, Elliott (Ed) (1978) Health services; their nature and organisation and the role of patients, doctors, nurses and the complementary professions. London: Heinemann.

Jefferys, Margot and Elliott, Patricia M (1966) Women in medicine. London: Office of Health Economics.

Jefferys, Margot; Millard, J B; Hyman, Mavis and Warren, M D (1969) 'A set of tests for measuring motor impairment in prevalence studies' Journal of Chronic Diseases 22 303–319.

Johnson, Gillian S and Johnson, R H (1977) 'Social-services support for multiple sclerosis patients in west of Scotland' Lancet 1 31–34.

Johnston, Lennox (1952) 'Aetiology of carcinoma of lung' (Correspondence) British Medical Journal 2 1417.

Jolleys, J C W; Barnes, R J and Gear, M W L (1978) 'A follow-up survey of patients with dyspepsia in one general practice' Journal of the Royal College of General Practitioners 28 747–751.

Jones, J Spencer (1981) 'Telling the right patient' British Medical Journal 283 291–292.

Journal of the Royal College of General Practitioners (1976) 'Looking after patients with high blood pressure' (Editorial) 26 235–236.

Joyce, C R B; Last, J M and Weatherall, M (1968) 'Personal factors as a cause of differences in prescribing by general practitioners' British Journal of Preventive and Social Medicine 22 170–177.

Kayser-Jones, Jeanie Schmit (1981) Old, alone, and neglected: care of the aged in Scotland and the United States. Comparative studies of health systems and medical care. University of California Press.

Kessel, Neil and Shepherd, Michael (1965) 'The health and attitudes of people who seldom consult a doctor' Medical Care 3 6–10.

Kiernan, K E (1977) 'Age at puberty in relation to age at marriage and parenthood: a national longitudinal study' Annals of Human Biology 4 301–308.

Kinsey, A C; Pomeroy, W B and Martin, C E (1948) Sexual behaviour in the human male. Philadelphia: Saunders.

Klein, Rudolf (1978) 'Brunel on a Cook's tour' British Medical Journal 2 1703.

Knight, R and Warren, M D (1978) Physically disabled people living at home: a study of numbers and needs. London: HMSO.

Kohn, Robert and White, Kerr L (Eds) (1976) Health care. An international study. London: Oxford University Press.

Lancet (1977) 'Incontinent women' Lancet 1 521–522.

Lancet (1981) 'Counting the dead is not enough' Lancet 2 131–132.

Lancet (1983) 'Confidentiality and accountability' Lancet 1 277–278.

Lee, J A H; Draper, P A and Weatherall, M (1965) 'Primary medical care: prescribing in three English towns' Milbank Memorial Fund Quarterly 43 285–290.

Lievesley, Denise; Breeze, Elizabeth and Owen, Delyth 'Postcode sampling' Office of Population Censuses and Surveys. Unpublished paper.

Lindsey, Almont (1962) Socialized medicine in England and Wales: the National Health Service 1948–1961. London: Oxford University Press; The University of North Carolina Press.

Logan, R F L (1964) 'Studies in the spectrum of medical care' In Problems and progress in medical care edited by Gordon McLachlan. London: Oxford University Press for Nuffield Provincial Hospitals Trust.

Logan, W P D and Brooke, Eileen M (1957) 'The survey of sickness 1943 to 1952' General Register Office Studies in Medical and Population Subjects No. 12. London: HMSO.

London Health Planning Consortium (1981) Primary health care in Inner London: report of a study group. London: DHSS.

Lorber, J (1971) 'Results of treatment of myelomeningocele. An analysis of 524 unselected cases, with special reference to possible selection for treatment' Developmental Medicine and Child Neurology 13 279–303.

Lorber, J (1972) 'Spina bifida cystica. Results of treatment of 270 consecutive cases with criteria for selection for the future' Archives of disease in childhood 47 854–873.

Lorber, John and Salfield, Stephen A W (1981) 'Results of selective treatment of spina bifida cystica' Archives of disease in childhood 56 822–830.

Lowdon, A G R; Stewart, R H M and Walker, W (1966) 'Risk of serious infection following splenectomy' British Medical Journal 1 446–450.

MacArthur, Christine (1981) 'Speed of diagnosis, referral and treatment in cancer of the breast and large bowel' Department of Epidemiology, University of Manchester. Report to DHSS.

Macintyre, Sally (1977) Single and pregnant. London: Croom Helm.

Macintyre, Sally (1980) 'Telling motherhood as it really is' Times Higher Educational Supplement 6 June 1980.

Macintyre, Sally (1981) 'Consumer reactions to ante-natal services' Paper given at conference on Pregnancy Care for the 80s – a challenge to the Profession, at Royal Society of Medicine.

McCance, C and Hall, D J (1972) 'Sexual behaviour and contraceptive practice of unmarried female undergraduates at Aberdeen University' British Medical Journal 2 694–700.

McCrossan, Liz (1979) 'Some suggestions for further experiments on interviewer coding of occupations' OPCS Survey Methodology Bulletin No. 5. p. 14.

McKee, Lorna and O'Brien, Margaret (Eds) (1982) The father figure. London: Tavistock.

McKee, W J E (1963) 'A controlled study of the effects of tonsillectomy and adenoidectomy in children' British Journal of Preventive and Social Medicine 17 49–69.

McKenna, S P; Hunt, S M and McEwan, J (1981) 'Weighting the seriousness of perceived health problems using Thurstone's method of paired comparisons' International Journal of Epidemiology 10 93–97.

McKeown, T (1973) 'A conceptual background for research and development in medicine' International Journal of Health Services 3 17–28.

McKeown, Thomas and Lowe, C R (1966) An introduction to social medicine. Oxford: Blackwell Scientific Publications.

McKinlay, John B (1970) 'The new late comers for antenatal care' British Journal of Preventive and Social Medicine 24 52–57.

McKinlay, Sonja M and Jefferys, Margot (1974) 'The menopausal syndrome' British Journal of Preventive and Social Medicine 28 108–115.

McKinlay, Sonja, Jefferys, Margot and Thompson, Barbara (1972) 'An investigation of the age at menopause' Journal of Biosocial Science 4 161–173.

Marmot, M G; Page, C M; Atkins, E and Douglas, J W B (1980) 'Effect of breast-feeding on plasma cholesterol and weight in young adults' Journal of Epidemiology and Community Health 34 164–167.

Marquis, Kent H and Cannell, Charles F (1971) Effect of some experimental interviewing techniques on reporting in the Health Interview Survey. Vital and Health Statistics Series 2 No. 41. Washington PHS.

Marsh, Geoffrey and Kaim-Caudle, Peter (1976) Team care in general practice. London: Croom Helm.

Martin, Jean and Monk, Janet (1982) Infant feeding 1980. London: OPCS.

Martin, J P (1957) Social aspects of prescribing. London: Heinemann.

Martini, Carlos J M; Allan, G J Boris; Davison, Jan and Backett, E Maurice (1977) 'Health indexes sensitive to medical care variation' International Journal of Health Services 7 293–309.

Mather, H G and others (1971) 'Acute myocardial infarction: home and hospital treatment' British Medical Journal 3 334–338.

Mawson, Stuart R; Adlington, Peter and Evans, Mair (1967) 'A controlled study evaluation of adeno-tonsillectomy in children' Journal of Laryngology and Otology 81 777–790.

Mechanic, David (1968) 'General practice in England and Wales: results from a survey of a national sample of general practitioners' Medical Care 6 245–260.

Mechanic, David (1972) 'General medical practice: some comparisons between the work of primary care physicians in the United States and England and Wales' Medical Care 10 402–420.

Medical Research Council (1957) 'Tobacco smoking and cancer of the lung. A statement' British Medical Journal 1 1523–1524.

Morgan, W; Walker, J H; Holohan, Ann M and Russell, I T (1974) 'Casual attenders: a socio-medical study of patients attending accident and emergency departments in the Newcastle upon Tyne Area. Hospital & Health Services Review June 1974 189–194.

Morrell, D C; Avery, Alison J and Watkins, C J (1980) 'Management of minor illness' British Medical Journal 280 769–771.

Morrell, D C; Gage, H G and Robinson, N A (1971) 'Symptoms in general practice' Journal of the Royal College of General Practitioners 21 32–43.

Morris, J N (1957) Uses of epidemiology. Edinburgh and London: E & S Livingstone.

Moser, C A and Kalton, G (1971) Survey methods in social investigation. London: Heinemann.

Moss, Louis and Goldstein, Harvey (Eds) (1979) 'The recall method in social surveys' Studies in Education 9, University of London, Institute of Education.

Murch, M (1980) Justice and welfare in divorce. London: Sweet and Maxwell.

National Opinion Poll (1980) Private treatment and private medical insurance as a job benefit. NOP Market Research Survey for BUPA.

Newton, K (1976) Second city politics: democratic processes and decision making in Birmingham. London: Oxford University Press.

Oakley, Ann (1979) Becoming a mother. London: Martin Robertson.

Oakley, Ann (1980) Women confined: towards a sociology of child birth. London: Martin Robertson.

Oakley, Ann (1981) 'Interviewing women: a contradiction in terms' In Doing feminist research edited by Helen Roberts. London: Routledge and Kegan Paul.

O'Brien, Maureen and Hodes, Charles (1979) 'High blood pressure: public views and knowledge' Journal of the Royal College of General Practitioners 29 234–239.

O'Brien, Maureen and Smith, Christopher (1981) 'Women's views and experiences of ante-natal care' The Practitioner 225 123–125.

Office of Population Censuses and Surveys, Social Survey Division (1973) The General Household Survey. Introductory Report. An inter-departmental survey sponsored by the Central Statistical Office. London: HMSO.

Office of Population Censuses and Surveys, Social Survey Division (1975) The General Household Survey 1972. London: HMSO.

Office of Population Censuses and Surveys, Social Survey Division (1976) General Household Survey 1973. London: HMSO.

Office of Population Censuses and Surveys, Social Survey Division (1978) The General Household Survey 1976. London: HMSO.

Office of Population Censuses and Surveys, Social Survey Division (1979) General Household Survey 1977. London: HMSO.

Office of Population Censuses and Surveys, Social Survey Division (1980) The General Household Survey 1978. London: HMSO.

Office of Population Censuses and Surveys, Social Survey Division (1981) General Household Survey 1979. London: HMSO.

Office of Population Censuses and Surveys, Social Survey Divisions (1982a) The General Household Survey 1979. London: HMSO.

Office of Population Censuses and Surveys (1982b) The General Household Survey 1980. London: HMSO.

Palmer, S R (1978) 'The use of mortality data in resource allocation' In Morbidity and its relationship to resource allocation edited by J H F Brotherston. Welsh Office.

Parish, Peter and Austin, Gay (1976) 'Prescribing repertoires of doctors new to general practice' In Prescribing in general practice. Journal of the Royal College of General Practitioners, Supplement 1, Vol. 26.

Parish, Peter A; Stimson, Gerry V; Mapes, Roy and Cleary, Jean (1976) Prescribing in general practice. Journal of the Royal College of General Practitioners 26 Supplement 1.

Parkhouse, J and McLaughlin, C (1976) 'Career preferences of doctors graduating in 1974' British Medical Journal 2 630–632.

Parkhouse, J and Palmer, M K (1977) 'Career preferences of doctors qualifying in 1975' British Medical Journal 2 25–27.

Parkin, D M; Henney, C R; Quirk, J and Crooks, J (1976) 'Deviation from prescribed drug treatment after discharge from hospital' British Medical Journal 2 686–688.

Parkin, D M; Kellett, R J; Maclean, D W; Ryan, M P and Fulton,

Mary (1979) 'The management of hypertension – a study of records in general practice' Journal of the Royal College of General Practitioners 29 590–594.

Patrick, Donald L (1981)) Health and care of the physically disabled in Lambeth. The longitudinal disability interview survey Phase 1 report. London: Department of Community Medicine, St Thomas' Hospital Medical School.

Patrick, Donald L; Darby, Sarah C; Green, Stephen; Horton, Geoffrey; Locker, David and Wiggins, Richard D (1981) 'Screening for disability in the inner city' Journal of Epidemiology and Community Health 35 65–70.

Patrick, D L; Peach, H and Gregg, I (1982) 'Disablement and care: a comparison of patient views and general practitioner knowledge' Journal of the Royal College of General Practitioners 32 429–434.

Peach, Hedley; Green, Stephen; Locker, David; Darby, Sarah and Patrick, Donald L (1980) 'Evaluation of a postal screening questionnaire to identify the physically disabled' International Rehabilitation Medicine 2 189–193.

Pearce, S; Knight, C and Beard, R W (1982) 'Pelvic pain – a common gynaecological problem' Journal of Psychosomatic Obstetrics and Gynaecology 1 12–17.

Peel, John and Carr, Griselda (1975) Contraception and family design. Edinburgh, London and New York: Churchill Livingstone.

Peterson, O L; Andrews, L P; Spain, R S and Greenberg, B G (1956) 'An analytic study of North Carolina general practice 1953–1954' Journal of Medical Education 31 No. 12, Part 2.

Platt, Jennifer (1978) 'Survey data and social policy' In Social Policy Research edited by Martin Bulmer. Macmillan.

Pless, Ivan Barry and Douglas, James W B (1971) 'Chronic illness in childhood: Part 1. Epidemiological and clinical characteristics' Pediatrics 47 405–414.

Porter, A M W (1969) 'Drug defaulting in general practice' British Medical Journal 1 218–222.

Pringle, M L Kellmer; Butler, N R and Davie, R (1966) 11,000 Seven year olds. London: Longman in association with National Children's Bureau.

Rantzen, Esther and Watts, Gordon (1982) 'That's life – having a baby' British Medical Journal 284 1049.

Raphael, W (1969) Patients and their hospitals. London: King's Fund.

Rashid, Aly (1982) 'Do patients cash prescriptions?' British Medical Journal 284 24–26.

Rayner, Claire (1981) 'Is your GP really good for you?' Woman's Own, 7 11 81.

Rayner, Claire (1982) 'You like your doctor but . . .' Woman's Own, 20 3 82.

Registrar General (1955) Statistical review of England and Wales for the two years 1950–51 Supplement on general morbidity cancer and mental health. London: HMSO.

Review Body on Doctors' and Dentists' Remuneration Twelfth Report – Appendix (1982) London: HMSO.

Ritchie, Jane; Jacoby, Ann and Bone, Margaret (1981) Access to primary health care. London: HMSO (OPCS Social Survey Division)

Rothschild, Lord (1971) 'The organisation and management of government R & D' In A framework for government research and development. London: HMSO. Cmnd. 4814.

Royal College of General Practitioners (1974) Morbidity studies from general practice. Second National Study 1970–71. Studies on medical and population subjects No. 26. London: HMSO.

Royal Commission on Medical Education 1965–68 (1968) Report. (Chairman: Lord Todd) London: HMSO. Cmnd. 3569.

Royal Commission on the National Health Service (1979) Access to primary care. Research paper number 6. London: HMSO.

Roydhouse, N (1969) 'A controlled study of adenotonsillectomy' Lancet 2 931–932.

Russell, I T (1977) 'British patients' choice of care for minor injury: a case study of separate sample logistic discrimination' 1977 Social Statistics Section. Proceedings of the American Statistical Association 548–553.

Russell, M A H; Wilson, C; Taylor, C and Baker, C D (1979) 'Effect of general practitioners' advice against smoking' British Medical Journal 2 231–235.

Sadler, J and Whitworth, T (1975) Reserves of nurses. An enquiry carried out on behalf of the Department of Health and Social Security. London: HMSO.

Sansom, C Dianne; MacInerney, Janet; Oliver, Valerie and Wakefield, John (1975) 'Differential response to recall in a cervical screening programme' British Journal of Preventive and Social Medicine 29 40–47.

Saunders, Cicely M S (1969) 'The moment of truth: care of the dying person' In Death and Dying edited by Leonard Pearson. Cleveland: Case Western Reserve University Press.

Schofield, Michael (1965) The sexual behaviour of young people. London: Longman.

Schofield, Michael (1973) The sexual behaviour of young adults. London: Allen Lane.

Scott, C (1961) Research on mail surveys. Social Survey Papers. Methodological Series No. 100.

Scott-Samuel, Alex (1981) 'Social class inequality in access to primary care: a critique of recent research' British Medical Journal 283 510–511.

Shanas, Ethel; Townsend, Peter; Wedderburn, Dorothy; Friis, Henning; Milhøj, Paul and Stehauver, Jan (1968) Old people in three industrial societies. London: Routledge and Kegan Paul.

Shands, H C; Finesinger, J E; Cobb, S and Abrams, Ruth D (1951) 'Psychological mechanisms in patients with cancer' Cancer 4 1159–1170.

Sheikh, K and Mattingly, S (1981) 'Investigating non-response bias in mail surveys' Journal of Epidemiology and Community Health 35 293–296.

Shepperdson, Billie (In press) 'Parents' views on abortion and euthanasia of Down's syndrome children'. Journal of Medical Ethics.

Simms, Madeleine (1981) 'Outlook for the Down syndrome child' Lancet 2 864.

Simms, Madeleine (1982) 'Teenage mothers by chance not choice' Family Planning To-day Second quarter.

Simms, Madeleine and Smith, Christopher (1982) 'Young fathers: attitudes to marriage and family life' In The father figure edited by Lorna McKee and Margaret O'Brien. London: Tavistock.

Simpson, Peter (1969) 'Teaching in family planning 1965–66' British Journal of Medical Education 3 84–93.

Slater, P (1946) Survey of sickness Oct 1943 to December 1945. The Social Survey.

Smith, Christopher (1981) 'How complete is the electoral register?' Political Studies 29 275–278.

Speak, Mary and Aitken-Swan, Jean (1982) Male midwives: a report of two studies. London: DHSS.

Stark, O; Atkins, E; Wolff, O H and Douglas, J W B (1981) 'Longitudinal study of obesity in the National Survey of Health and Development' British Medical Journal 283 13–17.

Statistical Office of The European Communities (1981) Qualitative survey of health, health services and housing in eight member countries of the European Communities – 1977. Luxembourg: Statistical Office of the European Communities.

Stimson, Gerry V (1976) 'Doctor patient interaction and some problems for prescribing' In Prescribing in general practice Journal of the Royal College of General Practitioners 26 Supplement No. 1.

Stocks, Percy (1947) 'Regional and local differences in cancer death rates.' General Register Office Studies in Medical and Population Subjects No. 1. London: HMSO.

Stocks, P (1949) 'Sickness in the population of England and Wales 1944–1947' General Register Office, Studies on Medical and Population Subjects No. 2. London: HMSO.

Taylor, Keith B (1982) 'Preventive medicine in general practice' British Medical Journal 284 921–922.

The Times (1981) 'Parents split over euthanasia for babies' 21 8 81.

Thomas, Thelma M; Plymat, Kay R; Blannin, Janet and Meade, T W (1980) 'Prevalence of urinary incontinence' British Medical Journal 281 1243–1245.

Thompson, Barbara; Hart, Shirley A and Durno, D (1973) 'Menopausal age and symptomatology in a general practice' Journal of Biosocial Science 5 71–82.

Titmuss, Richard M (1968) Commitment to welfare. London: Allen and Unwin.

Titmuss, Richard M (1970) The gift relationship: from human blood to social policy. London: Allen and Unwin.

Todd, G F (1975) Changes in smoking patterns in the UK. Tobacco Research Council Occasional Paper 1.

Townsend, Peter (1957) The family life of old people. London: Routledge and Kegan Paul.

Townsend, Peter (1962) The last refuge. London: Routledge and Kegan Paul.

Twining, T C and Chapman, J R (1980) 'Management of acute stroke in the elderly' British Medical Journal 281 1142.

Wadsworth, M E J; Butterfield, W J H and Blaney, R·(1971) Health and sickness: the choice of treatment. London: Tavistock.

Wadsworth, Michael (1979) Roots of delinquency. Oxford: Martin Robertson.

Wakefield, John and Baric, Leo (1965) 'Public and professional attitudes to a screening programme for the prevention of cancer of the uterine cervix. A preliminary study' British Journal of Preventive and Social Medicine 19 151–158.

Wakeley, Cecil (1964) 'Deaths from smoking' (Letter) British Medical Journal 1 1634.

Wandless, Irene; Mucklow, J C; Smith, Andrew and Prudham, D (1979) 'Compliance with prescribed medicines: a study of elderly patients in the community' Journal of the Royal College of General Practitioners 29 391–396.

Warren, M D (1975) Handicapped people in the community. A survey of agencies' records in Canterbury. University of Kent at Canterbury. Health Services Research Unit.

Warren, M D (1976) 'Interview surveys of handicapped people: the accuracy of statements about the underlying medical conditions' Rheumatology and Rehabilitation 15 295–302.

Waters, W H R; Gould, N V and Lunn, J E (1976) 'Undispensed prescriptions in a mining general practice' British Medical Journal 1 1062–1063.

Weale, Jane and Bradshaw, Jonathan (1980) 'Prevalence and characteristics of disabled children: findings from the 1974 General Household Survey' Journal of Epidemiology and Community Health 34 111–118.

Webb, Barbara and Williams, W M (1972) 'Mobility of general practitioners during the first few years in general practice' Sociological Review 20 591–600.

Weiss, C H (1977) 'Introduction' in Using social research in public policy making edited by C H Weiss. Farnborough: Saxon House.

Wilkes, Eric (1965) 'Terminal cancer at home' Lancet 1 799–801.

Willcocks, Dianne M; Cook, Jane; Ring, Jim and Kelleher, Robin (1980) PSS: Consumer study in old people's homes. Pilot report. Polytechnic of North London, Survey Research Unit, Dept. of Applied Social Studies, Research Report No. 6.

World Health Organization (1980) International classification of impairments disabilities and handicaps. Geneva: WHO.

Wright, Alastair F (1982) 'Sterilisation of women: prevalence and outcome' British Medical Journal 285 609–611.

Yarnell, J W G; Voyle, G J; Richards, C J and Stephenson, T P (1981) 'The prevalence and severity of urinary incontinence in women' Journal of Epidemiology and Community Health 35 71–74.

Zachary, R B (1977) 'Life with spina bifida' British Medical Journal 2 1460–1462.

Subject Index

Name index